# Understanding AIDS

# Understanding AIDS

## A Comprehensive Guide

### Edited by
### Victor Gong

Foreword by Mervyn F. Silverman

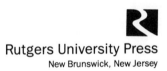

Rutgers University Press
New Brunswick, New Jersey

Library of Congress Cataloging in Publication Data
Main entry under title:
Understanding AIDS.
  Bibliography: p.
  Includes index.
    1. Acquired immune deficiency syndrome. I. Gong, Victor, 1956–  .  II. Title:
Understanding A.I.D.S. [DNLM: 1. Acquired Immunodeficiency Syndrome. WD
308 U55]
RC607.A26U53      1985        616.9        84–26233
ISBN 0–8135–1100–3
ISBN 0–8135–1101–1 (pbk.)

To my parents,
Alfred Kar Gong and Shun Yee Gong,
for without their love and support
this book could not have been written,
and to the memory of Dr. Peter Ho.

# Contents

# Foreword

It is hard for us today to understand the terrible fear of disease that haunted humankind throughout history. Advances in science and medicine over the past century have made us feel confident that the causes of disease will be found, cures established, and simple means of prevention developed. Doubts about modern medicine's effectiveness, raised by the new diseases Legionnaire's disease and toxic shock syndrome, were dispelled when medical researchers rather quickly identified the sources of these diseases and methods for controlling them.

Beginning in 1979, however, doctors became aware of a disease syndrome for which there was no known cause, no proven mode of transmission, and no cure. This disease, acquired immune deficiency syndrome (AIDS), seems to have originated in equatorial Africa and is thought to have migrated by some means to Haiti. It then appeared in New York City and, the following year, in San Francisco. It has since been seen in 45 states, Puerto Rico, Washington, D.C., and at least 30 other countries. As the number of cases increased, it became obvious that, whatever its origins, the disease predominantly afflicts bisexuals, homosexuals, and individuals who intravenously inject street drugs. The number of new cases in the United States began to rise at a rate that doubled every 6 months. This frightening situation shook public confidence in the medical profession and produced fear and frustration in both affected groups and the general population.

In 1981, we in San Francisco were facing one of the most complex health-care problems of the twentieth century. Homosexual and bi-sexual males represent approximately 20% of our population. Unlike in New York, AIDS cases in San Francisco were found almost exclusively in this group. While AIDS victims, their friends, and their families were overwhelmed by the realization that increasing numbers would suffer this illness and die prematurely, the rest of the community watched nervously, their response occasionally approaching hysteria. By the summer of 1983, we were faced with two epidemics: the tragic disease of AIDS and extreme anxiety in the general population. Paradoxically, the more we publicized our statistics and epidemiologic results that indicated AIDS was not spread through casual contacts, the higher the anxiety level rose. Courthouse clerks wondered if they were at risk for accepting a piece of paper from someone who might have AIDS; police wanted to wear gloves and masks when dealing with any member of the gay community. Other counties and states began to send their AIDS patients, sometimes in desperately ill condition, to San Francisco rather than give them appropriate care locally. This appeared to be due to fear of both contagion and financial cost. Telephones at the Health Department rang incessantly with calls from people wanting to know if they were in fact at risk for contracting this disease. The public was initially unwilling to accept the information being provided because it was based on experience with other illnesses none of which were universally fatal.

Intensive education and information programs, based on our most reasonable assumptions, significantly diminished unrealistic concerns within the general community, and energies were then concentrated more directly on providing necessary guidance to those most vulnerable so that they might remain free of this tragic disease. The effectiveness of this program was reflected in precipitously declining rates of sexually-transmitted non-AIDS diseases among homosexual and bisexual males, indicating a very significant decrease in the sexual behavior considered to enhance the risk for AIDS. Unfortunately, because of the long incubation period for AIDS, this has not yet been translated into a reduction in the incidence of new AIDS cases.

Over the past two years, a particular issue has constantly resurfaced and drawn the attention of politicians, the media, and the medical and legal professions. This issue deals with the existence of bathhouses, sex clubs, and other facilities that promote and profit from multiple, anonymous, unsafe sexual encounters among their patrons, and thus foster the spread of AIDS. Because a change in behavior throughout the high-risk community was our first priority, we felt that the initial requirements were a strong and effective educational program and a working partnership between the Health Department and the gay community. Action to regulate sex-related facilities would have reduced our chance for success, we thought, because it would not be recognized as necessary and would alienate those we needed most to reach. Furthermore, we feared such premature action would amount to an empty gesture because it was likely at that time to be overturned by the courts. By the spring of 1984, widespread changes in sexual behavior were taking place, the level of public knowledge about AIDS was high, and new scientific information suggested a definite association between attendance at these facilities and the spread of AIDS.

As Director of Health, I could no longer allow those facilities that encourage and facilitate the spread of AIDS to remain in operation. After failure of an approach using licensing regulation, the only course left open was to inspect these facilities and order closed those that were still encouraging unsafe practices. I had hoped that the gay community would take it upon itself to close the culpable businesses through community pressure, but unfortunately, this did not take place. Had it done so, it would have had an educational impact far greater than that of actions taken by the city government.

The bathhouse issue is especially significant insofar as it demonstrates the complexity of this disease in its various aspects: medical, social, ethical, political, and legal. Because of its many ramifications, the full impact of AIDS on society is difficult to anticipate. The central reality, and by far the most traumatic effect at this time, is that the lives of thousands of young men in their prime are being snuffed out because of AIDS. This fact alone demands understanding and compassion from us all. Simplistic solutions and the reactions of religious extremists have no place in dealing with this serious and complicated medical situation.

Regardless of research activities or regulatory government actions, education must continue to be the cornerstone of efforts to reduce the progression of the present epidemic. Only through intensive educational programs can we successfully prevent further dissemination of this fatal disease.

I believe this book will be a valuable tool in this regard. It provides an excellent compilation of what is known and what is postulated about AIDS. It offers useful information to health care providers and the general public, the worried well and those at minimal risk. One look at the table of contents indicates that the wide range of relevant issues has been covered; a reading of the chapters reveals that this is accomplished with considerable clarity, without sacrificing attention to the inherent complexities.

*Understanding AIDS: A Comprehensive Guide* presents us with an opportunity to arm ourselves with the knowledge essential in battling this disease and its devastating effects on our society.

MERVYN F. SILVERMAN

# Preface—Update on AIDS Research

AIDS (acquired immune deficiency syndrome) has not been out of the news since the syndrome was first described in 1981. Until quite recently, the headlines stressed its spread, its incidence in certain high-risk groups in the population, and its fearfully high mortality rate. Indeed, so little was known about the disease that even this kind of information was hard to establish.

Over the past two years, however, scientific and medical research into all aspects of AIDS has begun to yield insights into the nature of the disease, its cause, and possible means of treatment and prevention. In a remarkably short time we have made a start at understanding AIDS.

At the same time, though, we have come to realize more clearly just how serious a disease AIDS is and how difficult it is to combat. The number of deaths from AIDS continues to rise each year; there are signs that new groups may be at risk; and new practical and ethical questions about AIDS confront us as individuals and as a society.

While the contributors to this book have tried to make their discussions as up to date as possible, new research has been reported between the time of writing and the time the manuscript was sent to press. We have therefore added this summary of the most important new findings and developments as of the beginning of February 1985. In some cases, the research has not been formally published but announced through the news media.

The startling discovery and subsequent isolation and identification of the viral family responsible for causing AIDS has given scientists the tools needed to solve this medical dilemma. The culprit is a member of the retrovirus family, that is, viruses composed of genetic material called RNA (ribonucleic acid) instead of the more common DNA (deoxyribonucleic acid) found in most living things. The French physician Dr. Luc Montagnier claimed credit for identifying it in the lymph nodes of a homosexual male with the lymphadenopathy syndrome, and he termed the viral agent the "Lymphadenopathy Virus" or LAV. Dr. Robert Gallo of the National Cancer Institute shortly thereafter announced the American isolation of an almost identical virus, now known as Human T-cell lymphotrophic virus or HTLV-III. The two viruses proved later to be essentially the same.

This important achievement now allows drug companies to manufacture screening tests for the AIDS virus contaminating the nation's blood supply, to test drugs against the virus, and eventually to develop a vaccine. Epidemiologists are now able to study the disease in diverse segments of the population, to uncover the true spectrum of infection, and to learn more about the natural history and transmission of the AIDS virus.

Indeed, the new blood test that detects antibodies to the virus is already providing important information to medical investigators. The syndrome appears to be considerably more widespread than was thought. Large numbers of homosexuals, intravenous drug abusers, and hemophiliacs have antibodies to the AIDS virus in their blood, but show no symptoms of AIDS. This means that many people have been infected with the AIDS virus without having the classic symptoms of the syndrome. Extrapolating from the number of confirmed cases of AIDS, investigators estimate that 200,000 to 300,000 Americans may have antibodies to this virus in their blood. A positive blood test generally indicates that a person has encountered the virus. But researchers do not know if these individuals are immune to the disease, are "carriers," or will eventually develop the fullblown syndrome of AIDS.

Because the incubation period for AIDS is anywhere from several months to five years, the majority of infected adults will not show signs of the disease for a few years. Preliminary studies report that in groups of homosexual men who had antibodies to the virus in their blood two to five years ago, 5–19% have come down with

AIDS. Carefully planned studies are in progress to resolve these issues.

The AIDS blood test has other inherent limitations. A small number of patients may have a false-positive reaction (an error in the test that falsely indicates the presence of antibodies to the AIDS virus). But even more serious are false-negative tests, where individuals harboring the AIDS virus seem, according to this test, to be free of any AIDS antibodies.

A major dilemma for blood banks is what to tell the donor who has antibodies for the AIDS virus. The Centers for Disease Control (CDC) has published guidelines for administering these tests, and it recommends that people with positive tests be told that their prognosis is unknown at the present time, that they will probably remain infected, and that they can infect others. They are advised to refrain from donating blood, bodily tissues, or semen.

The costs for testing the approximately 12 million units of blood collected in the United States from 5 to 6 million donors will be substantial—perhaps 60 million to 120 million dollars annually. Medical counseling for donors found to have antibodies may be an even more costly burden to the blood bank system.

The advent of an AIDS screening test poses questions about patient confidentiality versus public health needs, inappropriate use of the test (i.e., as a surrogate test for homosexuality), and the potential denial of civil liberties to certain members of high-risk groups. However, the benefit of the test is clear; it will identify many asymptomatic carriers of the HTLV-III virus and will surely add an important measure of safety to the nation's blood supply.

In the United States, as of January 28, 1985, more than 8,000 cases of AIDS have been reported to the Centers for Disease Control; nearly half have already proved fatal. In this country, the groups at highest risk of contracting AIDS have not changed in the past five years: sexually active homosexual and bisexual men, intravenous drug users, recent Haitian immigrants, hemophiliacs, and female sexual partners of men with the syndrome. The proportion of cases not belonging to one of these risk groups has shown a minimal increase; the majority of these are due to blood product transfusions and a smaller number are due to sexual contact. However, a small but growing number of cases seem to involve sexually active heterosexual men and women. Heterosexual transmission of AIDS has been reported in both the United States and in Africa. However the number of such cases in the United States remains small, less than one percent of the total number of reported AIDS cases. When heterosexual transmission has occurred, it has been mainly from male intravenous drug abusers to their female sexual partners.

The growing concern that AIDS may be expanding its target group was spurred by recent findings about AIDS in several African countries. Interestingly, while the clinical features of the syndrome are the same in Africa as in America and Europe, the epidemiology of African AIDS offers striking contrasts. The two most important differences are the sex distribution and the apparent lack of risk factors. In Africa, men and women are afflicted with the syndrome in equal numbers, which suggests that transmission of AIDS occurs both from male to female and from female to male. In one study reported in *Lancet*, most of the African males with AIDS were promiscuous heterosexuals and some of the females were prostitutes. In all of the African AIDS cases, none of the patients admitted to homosexuality, intravenous drug abuse or blood transfusions. However, religious rituals and poor hygiene during medical procedures (i.e., using the same syringe on multiple patients) may play an important role in transmitting AIDS through blood. Further evidence of heterosexual transmission of AIDS in Africa comes from the unpublished cases of two separate clusters of AIDS involving males and females with frequent heterosexual contacts.

In the United States, the federal Centers for Disease Control report that about 4% of the 8,000 total AIDS cases belong to the category "noncharacteristic patients." These patients could not be classified into a group otherwise identified to be at increased risk for AIDS. Some of the men claimed to have frequent sexual contact with prostitutes. The role, if any, of female prostitutes in the heterosexual transmission of AIDS in the United States has not been established. Many of these prostitutes are intravenous drug users and could acquire the AIDS virus by this route. No one knows the actual incidence of infection in this group, but it is likely to be small. Future studies will clarify these unanswered questions about the role prostitutes may play in the transmission of AIDS.

Health care workers should take special note of information recently published by the CDC. The first report confirms the safety of the Hepatitis B vaccine. The vaccine is produced by pooled plasma of individuals with a prior hepatitis B infection, many of whom belong to the high-risk group for AIDS. Concern over the possibility that the AIDS virus might be present in the plasma and that it might survive the inactivation steps used to manufacture the vaccine has resulted in many healthcare workers avoiding vaccination. This study was unable to detect the virus or any of its products in the vaccine, and epidemiologic monitoring has failed to ascribe any AIDS cases to the vaccine.

The second study done by the CDC followed healthcare workers who had inadvertently exposed themselves to blood or bodily fluids of AIDS patients (i.e., through needlestick injuries, cuts with sharp instruments, contamination of open skin lesions, etc.). The study confirms that AIDS cannot be transmitted by casual contact, nor can it be spread through the air, and the risk of AIDS transmission by an accidental needlestick or other inadvertent contact with AIDS-infected materials is small, if any.

The prognosis still appears grim for the AIDS patient. Our armamentarium against the infections and cancers that kill these individuals has proved to be of limited value. Drugs like Bactrim and pentamidine are often used to treat *Pneumocystis Carinii* pneumonia (PCP), but are often ineffective and may even produce toxic reactions. A new drug called DFMO (difluoromethylornithine) has eradicated the PCP infection in six AIDS patients. We await further controlled studies to confirm the utility of this drug. Another drug, spiramycin, has proven to be effective in the treatment of cryptosporidiosis, a severe debilitating watery diarrheal disease. Also, aggressive combination chemotherapy has produced favorable responses in many cases of Kaposi's sarcoma.

Attempts to restore or at least boost the ailing body's immune system with agents like interferon and interleukin-2 have met with little success. Scientists are now directing their efforts at attacking the virus with antiviral agents and then trying to reconstitute the immune system. Ribavirin, a drug used in the treatment of other human viral infections, has been shown to suppress the reproduction of the AIDS virus in laboratory cultures. Clinical trials of this drug on human patients are pending.

The AIDS virus does have an unusual characteristic: it requires an enzyme called reverse transcriptase to infect and destroy white blood cells. An antiparasitic drug, suramin, used to treat African sleeping sickness, has shown promise by acting to inhibit the reverse transcriptase enzyme. This drug may be most useful in treating patients who show early signs of AIDS, before their immune system has been irreversibly damaged.

Dr. J.-C. Chermann of the Pasteur Institute recently announced the use of a drug called HPA-23, a compound made of antimony and tungsten, on an hemophiliac afflicted with an AIDS infection of the brain (toxoplasmosis). A year and a half after treatment, the patient had no relapse of the infection and showed no signs of the LAV virus. The drug works by inhibiting the enzyme reverse transcriptase (*Lancet*, February 1985).

The development of an AIDS vaccine would be society's best hope for preventing further epidemics. That task will prove to be a difficult one. No vaccine has ever been made against this family of viruses, so there is no experience to draw upon. Moreover, the HTLV-III virus has the ability to change its immunologic structure. In this, it is analogous to influenza, where different strains of the virus require the development of a new vaccine for each new strain. A vaccine that works against one strain of the HTLV-III virus will be of no use against another.

A more encouraging discovery is the existence of a "neutralizing antibody" found in the blood serum of people, both healthy and suffering from AIDS, who carry the HTLV-III virus. This "neutralizing antibody" seems to attach itself to the covering of the virus and to prevent the virus from infecting white blood cells. So far, this antibody has only been shown to stop the virus in laboratory experiments. Whether it can be equally effective in destroying the virus in the human body, and thus be used as a vaccine, remains to be seen.

More immediately hopeful is the announcement by the Mariposa Foundation and the CDC that a spermicide, nonoxynol-9, found in several commercially available contraceptives, can inactivate a strain of HTLV-III virus in the laboratory. It is not known whether the spermicide has the same effect in actual use on humans. It probably cannot hurt to use a spermicide containing nonoxynol-9 along with other precautions against the spread of AIDS, but no one should rely on it by itself for protection against the disease.

VICTOR GONG
February 1985

## REFERENCES

Anonymous. A new recruit against an opportunist killer. *Medical World News* 1985, Jan; 28:11–12

Broder S. and Gallo RC. A pathogenic retrovirus (HTLV-III) linked to AIDS. *N Engl J Med* 1984; 311:1292–1297

Brun-Vezinet F, Rodouzioux C, Montagnier L, et al. Prevalence of antibodies to Lymphadenopathy-associated retrovirus in African patients with AIDS. *Science*; 226:453–456

Centers for Disease Control. Antibodies to a retrovirus etiologically associated with acquired immunodeficiency syndrome (AIDS) in populations with increased incidences of the syndrome. *Morb Mortal Wkly Rep* 1984; 33:377–378

———. Hepatitis B vaccine: Evidence confirming lack of AIDS transmission. *Morb Mortal Wkly Rep* 1984; 33:685–686

———. Prospective evaluation of health-care workers exposed via parenteral or mucous-membrane routes to blood and bodily fluid of patients with acquired immunodeficiency syndrome. *Morb Mortal Wkly Rep* 1984; 33:181–182

———. Update: Acquired immunodeficiency syndrome (AIDS)–United States. *Morb Mortal Wkly Rep* 1984; 33:661–662

Chamberland ME, Castro KG, Haverkos HW, et al. Acquired immunodeficiency syndrome in the United States: An analysis of cases outside high-incidence groups. *Ann Intern Med* 1984; 101:617–623

Clumeck N, Sonnet J, Taelman H, et al. Acquired immunodeficiency syndrome in African patients. *N Engl J Med* 1984; 310:492–497

Goldsmith M. HTLV-III testing of donor blood imminent; complex issues remain. *JAMA* 1985; 253:173–181

McCormick JB, Mitchell SW, Getchell JP, et al. Ribavirin suppresses replication of lymphadenopathy-associated virus in cultures of human adult T lymphocytes. *Lancet* 1984; 1367–1369

Mitsuya H, Popovic M, Yarchoan R, et al. Suramin protection of T-cells in vitro against infectivity and cytopathic effect of HTLV-III. *Science* 1984; 226:172–174

Piot P, Quinn TC, Taelman H, et al. Acquired immunodeficiency syndrome in a heterosexual population in Zaire. *Lancet* 1984; 65–68

Portnoy D, Whiteside ME, Buckley E, et all. Treatment of intestinal cryptosporidiosis with spiramycin. *Ann Intern Med* 1984; 101:202–204

Ratner L, Haseltine W, Patarca R, et al. Complete nucleotide sequence of the AIDS virus, HTLV-III. *Nature* 1985; 313:277–283

Van de Perre V, Rouvroy D, Lepage P, et al. Acquired immunodeficiency syndrome in Rwanda. *Lancet* 1984; 62–64

Weiss SH, Goedert JJ, Sarngadharan MG, et al. Screening test for HTLV-III (AIDS agent) antibodies: Specificity, sensitivity, and applications. *JAMA* 1985; 253:221–225

# Acknowledgments

I would like to express deep appreciation to the many friends and colleagues who provided invaluable assistance during the preparation of this book. Thanks go to Ms. Ginna Briggs, for her assistance in the original copy editing, and the following friends who objectively reviewed the book: Evelyn Gong, Sherry Rush, Tina Green, Kathy Johnson, Joan-Cecelia Williams, Rose Mary Ryan, Mary Beth Thompson, Janet Netzke, Linda Masterson, Dr. Jeffrey Vieira, and Dr. Mervyn F. Silverman. Dr. Melvin Weinstein was very supportive and provided valuable insights. Special thanks to Rutgers University Press, Karen Reeds, and to Norman Rudnick for the final copy editing.

# Understanding AIDS

# One    The Twentieth Century Enigma

# 1     AIDS—Defining the Syndrome
## VICTOR GONG

## WHAT IS AIDS?

AIDS, an acronym for acquired immune deficiency syndrome, is an impairment of the body's ability to fight disease. It leaves the affected individual vulnerable to illnesses that a healthy immune system might overcome. The name appropriately defines the condition. It is *acquired*, that is, not inherited or genetic, but associated with the environment. *Immune* refers to the body's natural system of defense to combat disease, while *deficiency* indicates that the system is incomplete or lacking. A *syndrome* is a group of particular signs and symptoms that occur together and characterize a disorder.

AIDS patients are susceptible to diseases called opportunistic infections. These are illnesses due to organisms commonly found in the environment and harmful only to individuals with a weakened immune system. At first, AIDS patients feel as though they may have a cold, the flu, or some other viral illness. Their early symptoms, usually benign and inconspicuous, may include fatigue, loss of appetite, fever, night sweats, swollen glands (enlarged lymph nodes) in the neck, armpits, or groin, unexplained weight loss, diarrhea, persistent cough, and various skin lesions. However, these symptoms may persist for months or worsen as opportunistic diseases exploit the body's collapsed defenses. Many (52%) will develop an unusual pneumonia caused by the protozoan *Pneumocystis carinii*. Another third of these patients will exhibit a rare cancer of the skin, Kaposi's sarcoma (KS), or contract one of the many opportunistic diseases caused by fungi (yeast), viruses, bacteria, and protozoans.

Defining AIDS is difficult because there are no standardized criteria among clinicians and researchers to characterize the syndrome and its diagnosis. Some clinicians restrict the diagnosis only to patients who have developed serious infections, malignancies as e.g., KS, *P. carinii* pneumonia (PCP), or other opportunistic diseases. These are considered "markers" of AIDS, indicative of and specific for an underlying cellular immunodeficiency. The symptoms of these otherwise rare diseases are often the first signals of the development of AIDS. Other observers believe that only persistent laboratory evidence of immunodeficiency accompanied by the significant signs and symptoms listed in Chapter 4 is diagnostic of AIDS.

When should one suspect AIDS? AIDS should be suspected in patients under the age of 60 who develop recurrent or unusual infections under circumstances summarized in table 1. Such patients usually appear emaciated and have a history of prolonged (3 months or greater) fevers, night sweats, diarrhea, skin rash, and generalized swollen glands. Their personal history may include homosexuality or bisexuality, intravenous drug abuse, hemophilia, blood products transfusion, recent immigration from Haiti, or sexual contact with another AIDS patient. A child of any of the aforementioned groups is also susceptible. They are also free of other known causes of immunodeficiency such as cancers, malnutrition, treatments with steroids, radiation, or anticancer drugs, and have not had a recent viral illness such as measles or mumps. They also show laboratory evidence of a weakened immune state.

The Centers for Disease Control (CDC) in Atlanta, Georgia has proposed strict surveillance guidelines for physicians for the diagnosis of AIDS. Such guidelines will allow the CDC to obtain accurate data to detect disease patterns and monitor trends. The rigid nature of the CDC's guidelines, however, may not cover the wide clinical spectrum of AIDS and might result in an underestimate of the extent and severity of the problem. The guidelines portray one end of the spectrum and ignore milder forms of AIDS-related illnesses that may have less clearly defined clinical courses but greater prevalence in the general population. The entire spectrum of AIDS-related conditions is unknown but is thought to include a condition

**TABLE 1.   AIDS PATIENT PROFILE**

**Age**

Under the age of 60

**Personal History**

Homosexual and bisexual males
Intravenous-drug abusers
Recent Haitian immigrants
Hemophiliacs
Recipients of blood product transfusions
Sexual partners of patients with AIDS
Children of the above

**Past History**

No previous diseases or drugs (cancers, chemotherapy, steroids, malnutrition, recent viral illnesses) that might weaken immunity

**Symptoms**

Prolonged fevers
Severe weight loss
Persistent diarrhea
Skin rash
Persistent cough
Shortness of breath

**Signs**

Generalized swollen glands
Emaciation
Blue or purple-brown spots on the body, especially on legs and arms
Prolonged pneumonia

**Laboratory Data**

Tissue biopsy, sputum, blood, urine, etc., that confirm opportunistic infection or cancer
A low (less than 2) T-cell helper/suppressor ratio
Abnormal results in immunologic skin tests
Unexplained anemia (low blood count)

called lymphadenopathy syndrome (diffuse swollen glands), a variety of autoimmune diseases (illnesses due to an overactive immune system), and a generalized wasting syndrome. The CDC's data also omit children under the age of 5 who develop an AIDS-like clinical picture, which cannot be distinguished with certainty from diseases acquired during prenatal development. Nevertheless, most of such children have a parent with a history of intravenous-drug abuse or were born in Haiti, and a few have parents with AIDS. The CDC has recently created a provisional case definition for pediatric AIDS.

Thus, as its name states, AIDS is a syndrome, not a single disease or malignancy, with a broad clinical spectrum that ranges from severe infections and death to hidden disease states (i.e., carriers and recovered cases) and includes milder forms with possibly more hopeful prognosis.

## AIDS: THE SPECTRUM OF INFECTIONS AND MALIGNANCIES

AIDS victims are easy prey for a variety of viruses, bacteria, protozoans, and fungal pathogens that can cause single or multiple recurrent infections, collectively categorized as opportunistic (see table 2). All of us have pathogens in our body, e.g., herpes virus, chicken pox virus, candidal fungi (yeast), and even, occasionally, cancer cells, but our immune serveillance system normally prevents them from harming us. If our immunity is impaired or nonfunctioning, these pathogens seize the opportunity to spread destruction, so that the localized infection becomes widely disseminated or the single cancer cell multiplies and becomes a tumor (neoplasm). The immunodeficiency does not cause the mortality (death rate) and morbidity (sickness rate) of AIDS; rather, it creates the environment for opportunistic pathogens to do harm.

Most common in severely afflicted patients are PCP and KS, but a larger population of high risk groups may have a prodromal (early warning) or milder form of AIDS-related illnesses. It is important to appreciate this wide clinical spectrum to acquire a global view of the AIDS dilemma.

This broad range of disease states is not unique to AIDS. For example, when any susceptible host is exposed to an infectious source, the response may vary widely. At one extreme is infection that results

**TABLE 2.   COMMON DISEASES OR AGENTS OF INFECTIONS
IN AIDS PATIENTS**

| Viruses | Fungi | Protozoa |
|---|---|---|
| Herpesviruses | Candida | *Pneumocystis carinii* |
| (Types I and II) | Cryptococcus | *Toxoplasma gondii* |
| Cytomegalovirus | | Cryptosporidium |
| Varicella (chickenpox) | | *Giardia lamblia* |
| Adenovirus | | *Entameba histolytica* |
| Epstein-Barr | | |

**Bacteria**

Shigella
Salmonella
Campylobacter
*Neisseria gonorrhoeae*
Tuberculosis
(and atypical tuberculosis)
Syphilis

in death; at the other extreme is hidden or asymptomatic infection; in between are severe-to-mild illnesses from which the patients recover. Viral hepatitis B is a good example. Each year in the United States, about 200,000 persons, mostly young adults, acquire hepatitis B infections. The majority of cases are undetected (asymptomatic) or present with nonspecific complaints such as fatigue and nausea (the disease is often misdiagnosed as a flu-like illness). About 50,000 have symptomatic illness with nausea, vomiting, abdominal pain, and jaundice (yellow skin and eyes), but eventually recover; up to 20,000 (10%) then become carriers of the disease. Some 2,500 (1–2%) of infected persons die from liver failure and/or liver cancer.

The incidence of AIDS is similarly deceptive. Thus, AIDS disorders can be depicted as an iceberg: detected illness, above the water line, represents only a small proportion of the epidemic, while the majority of cases, below the water line, represent unapparent infections.

## Opportunistic Infections

*Pneumocystis Carinii Pneumonia*

PCP, the most common life-threatening opportunistic infection in AIDS patients, accounts for half of all diagnosed AIDS cases. The PCP protozoan parasite is found widely in the environment and in the lungs of animals and man. Because exposure to the organism has no serious consequences for healthy individuals with normal immune mechanisms, PCP is rare in the United States. Only recently has it been noted in severely malnourished infants, adults with such malignancies as leukemias and lymphomas (cancers of cells in the lymph nodes), patients undergoing chemotherapy that damages their immune systems, and organ transplant patients treated to suppress rejection of foreign tissue.

*Other Opportunistic Infections*

AIDS patients are easy prey for numerous other pathogens including other protozoans (e.g., toxoplasmosis and cryptosporidiosis), fungi (e.g., Candida), viruses (e.g., herpes, cytomegalovirus), and bacteria (e.g., tuberculosis, salmonella, amebiasis, etc.).

## Malignancies

*Kaposi's Sarcoma*

After PCP, KS is the second most common disease of AIDS patients. KS has been known as a rare malignant skin tumor that, prior to 1979, mainly affected elderly men of Mediterranean descent. Typically, it was limited to the skin, rarely affected other organs, and responded well to treatment. Patients often lived for 8 to 13 years after diagnosis and usually died of other diseases related to old age.

A more aggressive variety of KS, found in equatorial Africa, primarily strikes young men (usually before age 35), responds variably to treatment, and can spread to other organs. Recently, this type of KS is being seen in organ transplant recipients and cancer patients undergoing chemotherapy.

The KS seen in AIDS patients resembles the African variety. It predominantly affects young homosexual men and aggressively spreads to other organs besides the skin, including the lymph nodes, abdominal organs, and lungs.

*Other Malignancies*

In addition to KS, other rare malignancies implicated in AIDS include lymphomas and cancers of the skin, rectum, and mouth.

## CONDITIONS ASSOCIATED WITH AIDS

### Lymphadenopathy Syndrome

An individual diagnosed as having AIDS has already developed severe immunodeficiencies with consequent secondary infections and malignancies. There undoubtedly exist many others who have been infected but recovered, passing the ailment off as flu or not even noticing it. No one has succeeded in definitively identifying and observing AIDS in its primary stage, i.e., when the immune system is first attacked. Some researchers believe that a condition characterized by swollen glands and other nonspecific signs and symptoms may be a preliminary stage of AIDS. Many patients with AIDS recall having had generalized swollen glands (lymphadenopathy) for many months prior to their diagnosis.

In May of 1982, the CDC published reports indicating that an increasing number of cases of persistent, generalized swollen glands associated with fevers, malaise, night sweats, weight loss, and diarrhea had been observed in homosexual males. This was first termed the "Gay Lymphadenopathy Syndrome" but, since it has also been observed in other individuals at increased risk for AIDS, it is now more appropriately renamed simply the lymphadenopathy syndrome.

A patient is given this diagnosis if enlarged lymph nodes have appeared in at least two separate areas of the body (excluding the groin) for more than three months, no other cause is found, and a biopsied node shows nonspecific inflammation. Many conditions can cause lymphadenopathy, e.g., infections, especially viral such as mononucleosis, hepatitis, and cytomegalovirus, as well as bacterial such as tuberculosis and syphilis. Drugs, cancers, and autoimmune disorders may also cause lymph node swelling. These conditions must be excluded by appropriate laboratory studies and other tests before a diagnosis of lymphadenopathy syndrome is determined.

This condition appears to be related to AIDS in high-risk groups (homosexuals and drug users) who share many risk factors, e.g., sexual promiscuity and frequent use of recreational drugs. These individuals also have immunologic defects, such as low white blood cell count and inversion of the T-cell ratio, similar to those found in AIDS patients. But questions remain. Does the lymphadenopathy syndrome represent a prodromal or pre-AIDS state, or just a milder version of AIDS? Are these individuals at increased risk for developing AIDS?

Several studies are underway to answer these questions. It has been observed that the lymphadenopathy syndrome has sometimes progressed to classic AIDS and that infections or malignancies have developed, which suggests that it may be a prodrome or milder form of AIDS. In general, however, the outcome of these patients is not well defined. Preliminary studies offer conflicting results, one indicating that as many as 17% of these patients develop full-blown AIDS, while others show a much lower potential risk.

The lymphadenopathy syndrome creates a vexing clinical problem because so many diseases other than AIDS may cause similar signs and symptoms. On the basis of studies in progress, it can be said only that a small number of patients with this syndrome can be expected to acquire opportunistic infections and malignant diseases. Whether the underlying immune abnormalities in these patients are reversible also remains to be ascertained. The contribution of lifestyle, the natural course of the syndrome, and the relationship of the syndrome to AIDS require further investigation.

**Autoimmune Diseases**

Immunity is a protective system designed to be specific and discriminating in its surveillance of foreign intruders. The human immune system is able to discern the body's own cells and tissues (self) from alien cells and organisms (nonself). When this system malfunctions, the body indiscriminately attacks its own tissue by manufacturing antibodies directed against what it misperceives as foreign. The result is destruction of that tissue, a condition called autoimmunity. In AIDS, a similar disorder, idiopathic thrombocytopenic purpura (ITP), directs antibodies against the platelets, blood cells intimately involved in the clotting process. The destruction of platelets may produce no overt symptoms other than a reduced platelet count, but the consequences range up to an increased susceptibility to bruising or frank bleeding.

### The Wasting Syndrome

Some individuals at increased risk for AIDS develop a clinical picture of general debilitation associated with persistent weight loss (as much as 40%) over several months. They also have profound fatigue, diarrhea, and sometimes fever and swollen glands. Their cellular immunity is depressed, but not as severely as in AIDS patients. They may also develop one or more opportunistic infections.

### SUMMARY

The acronym, AIDS, the mystery of which is reflected in its cryptic name, is a label for a syndrome whose exact nature is the subject of considerable debate among physicians. The syndrome is seen in a select group of individuals at high risk and includes a variety of opportunistic infections and malignancies. However, many illnesses associated with this syndrome (e.g., autoimmune disorders, lymphadenopathy syndrome, and the wasting syndrome) have no clearly defined role and await further studies to reveal their relationship to AIDS. Since a diagnosis of AIDS places a devastating label on any patient, a strict definition should always be used. However, knowledge of the epidemiology and natural course of the disease is still evolving so that diagnostic criteria must continually be reevaluated as new information becomes available.

# 2     Assembling the AIDS Puzzle: Epidemiology

### KEEWHAN CHOI

In the late spring of 1981, Dr. Michael S. Gottlieb, four of his colleagues at the UCLA School of Medicine, and Dr. I. Pozalski at Cedars Mt. Sinai Hospital in Los Angeles came upon a remarkable medical mystery. Between October 1980 and May 1981 they treated 5 young male homosexuals hospitalized with *Pneumocystis carinii* pneumonia (PCP), a rare infection. All also had other "opportunistic" infections, normally seen only in organ transplant patients whose immune systems have been broken down intentionally to assist in acceptance of the new organ, and two of the men died during treatment. The sudden appearance of these diseases in so many otherwise healthy men was alarming. The doctors reported the cases in the June 5, 1981 issue of the Morbidity and Mortality Weekly Report (MMWR), published by the Centers for Disease Control (CDC), in Atlanta, Georgia, a periodical in which current public health problems and statistics are discussed.

At about the same time, Dr. Alvin Friedman of New York University called the CDC about an unusual number of cases of Kaposi's sarcoma (KS) he had found at New York University Hospital that past winter. Dr. Friedman and his colleagues reported in the July 3 issue of MMWR that 20 cases of KS had been discovered in New York and 6 in California in the 30 months from January 1979 to July 1981. All

26 were homosexual males, their ages ranging from 26 to 51; 4 also had PCP. Within 2 years after diagnosis of KS, 8 were dead. While this information was being digested, word came from California that 10 new cases of PCP had been identified. Again all involved homosexual men, and 2 also had KS. Concerned about these startling developments, the CDC, the federal agency responsible for controlling and preventing disease in the United States, formed a task force headed by Dr. Jim Curran that started a systematic search for cases of this as yet unnamed syndrome. They began looking for laboratory-proven cases of KS or opportunistic infections such as PCP in previously healthy people of either sex between the ages of 15 and 60. The target areas were chosen to include cities with varying proportions of homosexual men. The task force first contacted physicians, major hospitals, and tumor registries in New York State, California, and Georgia. The investigators also reviewed physicians' requests for pentamidine, a drug available only from the CDC and used to treat PCP. Later, the task force solicited detailed reports from physicians and health departments.

This early investigation went back to what the task force decided was probably the first case of the strange syndrome, one involving KS in New York City in 1978, and led to the conclusion that they were probably hunting down a totally new phenomenon. The next step was interviews with as many patients as possible to try to find out what was happening to homosexual men that was apparently not happening to anyone else. Dr. Harold Jaffe and other members of the task force went to San Francisco and New York to interview about 30 patients who were still alive. They conducted in-depth interviews about the patients' lifestyle, including homosexual behavior, drug use, and medical history.

It was quickly discovered that almost all of the patients regularly used "poppers"—amyl and butyl nitrites—as sexual stimulants. A theory was proposed that prolonged use of these nitrites might cause the new syndrome. The investigators focused on this and, within a few weeks, interviewed 416 homosexual and heterosexual men. It was quickly confirmed that use of the poppers was almost exclusively homosexual and that the heaviest users also tended to have the greatest number of sexual partners. Purchase and laboratory examination of the nitrites, however, failed to show whether the drugs could cause the new syndrome.

At this time, the fall of 1981, only 4 living heterosexual patients had been reported. Frustrated thus far, the task force designed in September a "case-control" study to seek possible causes of the syndrome in previously healthy young homosexuals. The study attempted to identify risk factors by comparing various characteristics of patients—cases—with those of healthy homosexual men—controls—with the hope of finding clues that would lead to the cause of the disease.

Using 20-page questionnaires, the investigators interviewed, in October and November of 1981, 50 homosexual victims of the syndrome and 120 healthy homosexual men, located through private physicians or venereal disease clinics in New York, San Francisco, and Los Angeles. The subjects were questioned for 60 to 90 minutes on their medical history, occupation, travel, exposure to toxic substances, use of both prescription and illegal drugs, use of inhalant sexual stimulants (poppers), sexual history, and family history. At the end of these interviews, the subjects, both cases and controls, were asked to donate biological specimens for laboratory comparisons. The task force took nearly a year to analyze the data from these sessions, using computers and sophisticated mathematical methods. They spent hundreds of hours discussing their project, from the design of the study and the questionnaire to the interpretation of results.

The most obvious difference between the cases and the controls, the study showed, was that men suffering from the new syndrome (the patients) tended to have many more sexual partners, an average of 60 per year, compared to 25 per year for the healthy homosexuals. The patients also were more likely to have frequented bathhouses, a common meeting ground for anonymous homosexual encounters. Other seemingly significant differences included a patient history of syphilis and non-B hepatitis and more common use of drugs such as marijuana and cocaine. The use of poppers, however, appeared to be the same for both cases and controls, casting doubt on the nitrites as a cause of the new syndrome. Laboratory studies by CDC virologists, microbiologists, and immunologists of the specimens obtained from the cases and controls were pursued to determine the character and extent of the breakdown of the immune systems in patients and to search for common or variant characteristics that might yield clues to the cause of the disease.

The patients were found to have a deficiency of T-helper cells, a type of white blood cell that assists the immune system in repelling invaders. Patients had elevated levels of IgG and IgA (proteins called immunoglobulins that are made in response to infection), higher titers of antibody to Epstein-Barr virus and cytomegalovirus, and a higher prevalence of antibody to hepatitis A. The chief conclusions of the study were that the disease could be transmitted through blood or semen, that the patients tended to have regular and anonymous sexual contacts in bathhouses, bars, and public restrooms, and that they engaged in sexual practices that produce abrasions and expose them to small amounts of blood, semen, and feces. The study also resulted in a name for the disease—acquired immune deficiency syndrome, or AIDS. Even as the task force was conducting its long investigation, AIDS was turning up in other segments of the population.

In the fall of 1981, Dr. Gerald Friedland of Montefiore Hospital in the Bronx, New York City, reported he had treated several cases of PCP and other opportunistic infections in heterosexual men and women. Their common connection was intravenous drug use. Health departments in New York and New Jersey reported that a small number of inmates in state prisons had similar symptoms. Physicians began reporting a new phenomenon, a wasting disease called lymphadenopathy, which they suspected might be an early stage of AIDS. The CDC task force dispatched more epidemiologists to investigate these patients.

Meanwhile, doctors at Jackson Memorial Hospital in Miami, Florida, told the CDC that autopsy reports showed that 4 Haitian immigrants had died of opportunistic infections. A few months later, they found similar infections among several other Haitians who had recently immigrated to the United States. This added a further intriguing facet to the medical mystery. Sexually active homosexual men and intravenous drug abusers might have habits in common that could expose them to the disease, but there was apparently little they could have in common with Haitian immigrants who, it seemed, were neither homosexual nor drug users.

The CDC sent Dr. Harry Haverkos to Miami to investigate the

Haitian cases, a difficult assignment because of the cultural and linguistic barriers. Haverkos tried to concentrate on what could have exposed the Haitians to AIDS. Reports reaching the CDC from Haiti, either from local physicians or from United States doctors visiting the island nation, indicated that both PCP and KS had been found among the natives.

By July, 1982, 10 months after the CDC first learned of the disease, there were 216 cases. Of those, 84% were homosexual men, 9% were intravenous-drug abusers, 2% were Haitians, and 5% were women; 88 of the patients were dead.

There had to be a common cause. Some still favored poppers, others suggested a new virus that attacked the immune system, and others favored an "immune-overload" theory. However, the Haitians remained the wild card, as they did not fit into any of the theories. Some investigators even doubted that the different groups had the same disease.

Drs. Curran, Jaffee, and others leaned toward the virus theory, and two events early in 1982 strengthened their suspicions. In January, the CDC discovered that a hemophiliac had died of PCP in Miami. However, the victim had received steroids, which weaken the immune system, had liver disease, and was dead, so the case was rejected as not fitting the CDC definition of AIDS. Then, in the spring, 2 more cases were reported, and their symptoms were similar to those of homosexual males, heterosexual intravenous-drug addicts, and recent Haitian immigrants suffering from AIDS. The most likely, and frightening, way that these hemophiliacs could have been exposed to AIDS was through the transfusions of clotting factors on which their lives depend.

Hemophiliacs lack part of a blood-clotting protein called Factor VIII, which must be replaced with injections derived from donor blood. A single injection can contain Factor VIII from 2,500 donors, thus exposing a hemophiliac to the blood of as many as 75,000 people every year. It appeared that whatever causes AIDS had gotten into the Factor VIII injections.

The July 16, 1982 issue of the CDC's MMWR reported that "the occurrence among the three hemophiliac cases suggests the possible transmission of an agent through blood products." In July, the U.S. Food and Drug Administration, the National Hemophiliac Foundation, and other organizations set up studies to evaluate the risks to hemophiliacs, examine Factor VIII supplies for contamination, and try to find ways of making the injections safer. By December 1982, the 3 original hemophiliac AIDS patients were dead, and 4 more heterosexual hemophiliacs had developed opportunistic infections and symptoms of a collapsed immune system. Intensive investigations into their sexual habits, drug usage, travel, and general lifestyle failed to produce any evidence that their disease could have been acquired through contact with each other, homosexuals, drug abusers, or even Haitian immigrants. There was one common link—all had received Factor VIII concentrate.

If the hemophiliac AIDS patients made the infectious organism theory likely, the discovery of the "LA cluster" made it more so. In February 1982, Dr. Jaffee and Dr. David Auerbach, the CDC officer in Los Angeles, heard rumors that some of the gay AIDS victims in the Los Angeles area had sexual contact with each other before they fell ill. Dr. Auerbach and Dr. Bill Darrow, a task force sociologist, began intensive interviews of the gay population of Los Angeles and were able to establish positive links between 9 of the 19 cases known in the area at the time. These homosexual men had had sexual relations with others in the group prior to their developing AIDS. Subsequent investigation enabled the task force to trace sexual connections among 40 patients in 10 cities.

A virus thus became the most likely culprit. It fit all the requirements—something transmitted sexually, especially through abrasions, carried by dirty needles, picked up in unsanitary living conditions, and able to contaminate blood. All of this was reminiscent of hepatitis B, the viral liver disease transmitted by blood, semen, or even saliva. However, there had been no evidence that, like hepatitis B, AIDS could be transmitted to anyone exposed to blood and blood products, receiving blood transfusions, or treated with dialysis machines.

Then, late in the fall of 1982, the task force was tracing down reports of children who might be suffering AIDS when they heard of a 20-month-old boy in San Francisco with symptoms of the disease. They learned that the boy had received transfusions and that one of the 19 donors was an AIDS patient they had interviewed in March. The donor had not had symptoms of the disease when he donated the blood. The CDC was later able to confirm that 2 adults had contracted AIDS after receiving blood transfusions, and 5 more hemophiliacs, including a 7-year-old and a 10-year-old, are believed to have the disease.

On January 4, 1983, representatives of every government health agency and commercial blood banks met in Atlanta to discuss ways of testing blood donors to screen AIDS carriers out of the system. Proposals included tightening federal regulations on commercial blood centers, banning donations from homosexuals or Haitians, and screening donors for a history of hepatitis B on the assumption that anyone who has had that disease might be more susceptible to AIDS. No decisions were made, and none of the proposals could be adopted without considerable opposition.

The CDC task force has opened files on two new victim groups—female sexual partners of men with AIDS, and children. By January 1983, 26 children under 5 years of age appeared to have contracted AIDS, and 10 were already dead. Although none had KS, all had PCP or similar opportunistic infections. Most of these victims were the children of Haitians, of intravenous drug users, or of men who had homosexual contacts. There is no indication how the children might have acquired the disease. More intensive pursuit of the disease in the United States and Puerto Rico turned up 2,259 cases by late 1983, some 80% concentrated in the metropolitan areas of New York, San Francisco, Miami, Newark, Houston, and Los Angeles. The progression of the investigation was paralleled by the increasing rate at which cases were reported—58 before 1981, 231 in 1981, 883 in 1982, and at least 1,087 in 1983. The incidence of AIDS has roughly doubled every 6 months since the second half of 1979. In September 1983, new cases were coming in to the CDC at the rate of 5 to 6 a day, as opposed to 2 a day in September 1982.

In 4 years, the reported number of AIDS cases increased to well over 3,000 in the United States and nearly 300 in Europe, mostly in England, West Germany, France, and Belgium, according to the World Health Organization and the Danish Cancer Society. (The total is now over 6000.) One way in which European AIDS cases differ from those in the United States is in their possible connection to Central Africa. About a quarter of the European cases are Africans and all of the first 40 Belgian cases had either lived in Central Africa

(Zaire or Chad) or had sexual contact with Central African residents. Also, African AIDS cases in Europe include about as many heterosexual men and women as homosexuals, so that homosexuality does not seem to be a factor among them.

A team of investigators from the CDC and the U.S. National Institutes of Health has found a substantial number of AIDS patients in urban hospitals in Zaire, but it is not known whether AIDS existed in Central Africa before appearing in the United States. The study of AIDS in Europe and Central Africa may provide clues to both its origin and pattern of transmission.

Over 40% of the AIDS victims found thus far have died. Deaths are due primarily to rare infections that a normal immune system easily controls. Among the many opportunistic diseases that attack AIDS patients, PCP appears to be the most deadly, accounting for 52% of the deaths. About 26% of AIDS patients have KS without any sign of PCP; 7% have both.

AIDS respects no racial or ethnic boundaries—57% of the cases are white, 26% are black, and 14% are Hispanic. Sex also offers no sure protection—147 victims have been women. The average patient age at diagnosis is 34; almost 47% are between 30 and 39, 22% are between 20 and 29, and another 22% are between 40 and 49. The ages of drug abusers with AIDS clustered more tightly—81% are between 20 and 39. Haitian victims tend to be even younger—47% are 20 to 29. Patients whose only apparent source of infection was blood transfusions tend to be older than 50.

The high-risk groups remain the same. Most cases (71%) are sexually active homosexual or bisexual men. The second largest group (17%) are heterosexuals addicted to intravenous drugs such as heroin and, like sexually active homosexual men, are known to have a high incidence of hepatitis B spread through the sharing of dirty needles. The third group, recent Haitian immigrants who are neither homosexual nor intravenous drug abusers, comprise 5% of the AIDS patients. About 1% of AIDS victims are hemophiliacs who are not homosexual and have no history of drug abuse or a Haitian background; 3% have no known common characteristics.

The most important link among all groups of AIDS victims is the peculiar breakdown of the immune system, which is evidently not a genetically acquired phenomenon. Most investigators have come to the conclusion that AIDS is caused by an infectious agent, probably a virus. Various viral candidates have been considered. For example, the spread of AIDS parallels that of hepatitis B. However, there is no evidence that hepatitis viruses are causing AIDS. Herpesviruses are among those that cause persistent infections of various body cells, and those herpesviruses that infect lymphocytes, notably the Epstein-Barr virus and cytomegalovirus, meet some of the criteria required of the agent that causes AIDS. Human T-cell leukemia virus (HTLV) is also transmitted from person to person, infects individuals in clusters, and is associated with the development of cancer over a long period. Although HTLV is not prevalent in the United States, scientists are searching for any role it may play in the development of AIDS. It is even speculated that the cause of AIDS may be a mutation, a virus from another species that has adapted to and spread among humans, or a virus that has long existed in a circumscribed human population where, for some reason, it did not receive specific medical attention.

The intense search for the cause, and ultimately the cure, of AIDS continues at the CDC and elsewhere around the world. For example, since some researchers suspect that patients with the vague syndrome called lymphadenopathy may actually be displaying an early stage of the disease, the task force is following the progress of such patients to learn if AIDS does indeed develop.

In the CDC laboratories, researchers put samples of urine, blood, sputum, and semen in cultures, examine the cultures under the electron microscope for foreign organisms, and isolate well-known viruses to inspect them for new or different characteristics. They also inject marmoset monkeys, chimpanzees, and mice with samples taken from patients to determine if the animals contract AIDS.

Although the above account dwells primarily on the CDC, the CDC is only one of many agencies involved in the search for the cause of AIDS. The U.S. Public Health Service (PHS) considers AIDS the number one health problem and has launched a multifaceted investigation, mostly through the CDC, the National Institutes of Health, the Food and Drug Administration, and the Alcohol, Drug Abuse and Mental Health Administration. These four PHS agencies spent 29 million dollars on AIDS work in 1983 and are scheduled to spend another 48 million in 1984. The investigation has also involved many scientists at universities and research institutes throughout the world.

Some promising results have appeared. In April 1984, a French team headed by Dr. Luc Montagnier at the Pasteur Institute in Paris isolated the lymphadenopathy virus (LAV) in 6 AIDS patients and in 5 lymphadenopathy patients. A team of researchers under Dr. Robert Gallo of the National Cancer Institute has found a new form of HTLV in AIDS patients, which they suggest as a possible cause of the disease. Tests must now be performed to clarify the relationship of these viruses to AIDS and also whether they are two distinct entities or actually the same single virus.

Meanwhile, the puzzle of AIDS is not yet solved and the search goes on.

# Two

# The Clinical Spectrum

# 3    The Immunology of AIDS
## HELEN L. LIPSCOMB

The human body is constantly bombarded by a variety of micro-organisms such as bacteria, viruses, fungi, and protozoans. How-ever, of the many thousands, only a few, perhaps 100 or so, cause disease in humans. Microorganisms that infect and cause disease in humans are called pathogens. When a pathogen enters the body, se-rious illness and often death may result unless the body has some means of protection.

The human body has developed two special mechanisms to cope with foreign invaders. The first, called innate immunity, is a non-specific mechanism present from birth that may be effective against all invaders. The second, called acquired immunity, or the immune system, is a very specific defense mechanism that depends upon proper functioning of the immune system of the body. Persons with the acquired immune deficiency syndrome (AIDS) have, for reasons not completely known at present, lost the ability to cope with for-eign invaders and are extremely susceptible to diseases caused by pathogens.

The purpose of this chapter is to discuss the changes known to oc-cur in the immune system of persons with AIDS. However, it is nec-essary to understand how the normal immune system works before it is possible to understand how it can malfunction. The first part of this chapter will explain how the normal, intact immune system operates. The next section will describe some of the better-known disorders of immunity. The last part of the chapter will concentrate on specific changes that occur in the immune system of patients with AIDS.

## THE NORMAL IMMUNE SYSTEM

Innate, nonspecific immunity includes protection provided by the skin, mucous membranes, and special chemicals within the body. The skin is a mechanical barrier that prevents foreign invaders from entering the body. The respiratory system contains a special lining composed of a mucus-secreting membrane whose cells carry tiny hairlike projections called cilia. The cilia are constantly moving and sweep foreign invaders, as well as other substances trapped in the mucus, out of the respiratory system. When the action of the cilia is impaired, for example, by cigarette smoke or the taking of certain types of drugs, increased susceptibility to respiratory infections may result.

Various secretions of the body also are important defenders against infection. Tears contain chemicals that attack bacteria, and stomach acids may kill many microorganisms that enter the stomach with food.

If microorganisms do gain entrance to the body, for example, through a break in the skin barrier, chemicals in the blood may destroy them. If these pathogens enter the body in sufficient numbers, a second line of defense, the immune system, is activated. This system is very specific for each type of microorganism it encounters, and immunity to a particular type develops only after exposure to that microorganism. Acquired immunity is normally lifelong. For example, when a child is first exposed to a measles virus, the immune system then becomes programmed to recognize and destroy the measles virus whenever it enters the body after the initial illness. Because of the specificity of the acquired immunity, exposure to measles virus does not provide protection against mumps, chickenpox, or any other infectious agent.

## ANATOMY OF THE IMMUNE SYSTEM

The immune system is complicated, and our understanding of its structure and function is far from complete. White blood cells, called lymphocytes, circulate throughout the body in the bloodstream. In addition to the bloodstream, there is another circulatory system called the lymphatic system. Collections of lymphocytes called lymph nodes (glands), connected to vessels of the lymphatic system, are located at strategic points throughout the body. Lymphocytes can leave blood vessels, travel through tissues and between cells of the body, enter the lymphatic system, and eventually return to the blood-stream. In this way, the lymphocytes patrol the body for foreign invaders. For example, if microorganisms get into body tissues through a cut in a finger, they are shuttled to lymph nodes in the elbow and axilla (armpit) where they are recognized and dealt with by lymphocytes. This prevents the microorganisms from multiplying and spreading throughout the body to cause generalized disease.

The immune system itself is divided into two parts—the cellular and the humoral immune systems. Cells of the cellular system are called T cells, and cells of the humoral system are called B cells. T cells receive their name from the thymus gland, located in the chest just above the heart. The thymus gland can be thought of as a learning center. It is responsible for processing and giving functional ability to lymphocytes, which come from the bone marrow. It also produces chemicals called thymus hormones, which circulate throughout the body and help regulate T-cell function.

A lymphocyte becomes a T cell by passing through the thymus gland. T cells are the controllers and regulators of the immune system. They recognize structures called antigens, which are present on microorganisms, and become programmed to respond to these antigens whenever they are encountered in the future. Recognition of antigens is very specific, and each T cell can recognize and respond to only one type of antigen. T cells also are the teachers of B cells and assist them in making chemicals called antibodies—such T cells are called helper T cells. Antibodies made by B cells can in turn attach to and kill microorganisms. Each antibody is also very specific and can react only with the particular antigen for which it was made. Another subpopulation of T cells, called suppressor T cells, regulates the amount of antibody made by B cells. This is important to ensure that B cells will not continue to make antibody when it is not needed.

B cells also originate in the bone marrow, and their main responsibility is to make antibody. Mature B cells circulate throughout the body. Once a B cell interacts with and is instructed by a T cell to make antibody, it develops into a plasma cell, the cell type that actually makes and secretes antibody. The antibodies are called immunoglobulins, or Igs.

There are 5 different types, or classes, of antibody that can be made by plasma cells. All have the same basic structure, but differ in size, location, and function. They are called IgG, IgA, IgM, IgE, and IgD. IgG makes up about 80% of the antibodies that circulate in the bloodstream and is important because it is produced in response to most infections. IgG can also cross the placenta and provide immunity to babies for up to 5 or 6 months.

IgM is actually the antibody produced upon first exposure to an infectious agent (primary immune response). However, upon subsequent exposure, B cells make IgG instead of IgM (secondary immune response). IgA is part of what is called the secretory immune system and is an important part of saliva and other secretions of the gastrointestinal tract. IgE is one of the factors involved in allergic reactions. The function of IgD is not known for certain.

There are other types of cells associated with immune responses. Macrophages ("large eaters") are cells that circulate throughout the body and search for foreign invaders. When they recognize such intruders, they communicate the information to T cells, which may then either kill the invaders or direct B cells to make specific antibody. Macrophages can also themselves engulf and destroy certain types of microorganisms.

Natural killer (NK) cells are another important type of cell involved in the immune system and have both specific and nonspecific functions. NK cells recognize cells of the body infected with virus and can nonspecifically kill these cells, thus preventing further production and release of virus. They can also recognize and kill certain types of tumor cells; for this reason, they are sometimes called the first line of defense against foreign virus and tumor attack. The origin of NK cells is not clear. Some scientists believe they may be a subpopulation of T cells, while others think they may be another type of lymphocyte.

Other cells of the body that act nonspecifically in defending against infection include white blood cells called polymorphonuclear leukocytes. These are somewhat similar to macrophages because they also can engulf and destroy foreign organisms.

## WHAT CAN GO WRONG WITH THE IMMUNE SYSTEM?

Because the immune system is complex, many parts may malfunction. In general, immune system problems can be divided into two general categories: inherited or congenital defects, and acquired defects. These defects may either enhance or depress immune responses. Inherited or congenital defects are present at birth, caused either by genetic errors or abnormal embryonic development. The "bubble baby" was a child born without an immune system, and thus no defenses against foreign invaders, who had to be physically isolated from sources of infection. Some children are born without a thymus gland and are very susceptible to infection by certain types of fungi and viruses. Other children have no B cells and cannot make antibodies against many types of bacteria. The immune system can also become overactive, resulting in autoimmune disease, the body's attack on its own tissues or cells.

### Inherited or Congenital Defects in Immune Function

*Primary Immune Deficiencies*
Instances of primary (congenital or inherited) immune deficiency are rare, but serious. T cells, B cells, or a combination of both may be involved. Also, some primary immune deficiencies affect other parts of the immune system, such as complement or macrophages.

In primary B-cell immunodeficiency, a child is unable to make antibodies and is especially susceptible to infection by bacteria. This is usually not noticed until a child is 5–6 months old because antibodies from the mother can cross the placenta, enter the baby's circulatory system before birth, and protect the child for several months after birth.

Primary T-cell immunodeficiencies are, fortunately, extremely rare. They are almost always associated with a problem in making antibody because nearly all antigens need both T and B cells for antibody production. Congenital thymic aplasia (DiGeorge's syndrome) is caused by abnormal embryonic development. A thymus gland either develops only partially or does not develop at all. In this disease, children are especially susceptible to infections from viruses and fungi.

Severe combined immunodeficiency (SCID) is a genetic disease that makes children especially susceptible to *Pneumocystis carinii*, cytomegalovirus (CMV), and Candida (thrush) infections. (These are also the three types of opportunistic infections most often seen in patients with AIDS.) Children with SCID are also vulnerable to many other types of bacterial and viral infections. The basic defect in SCID is thought to be a failure of stem cells from the bone marrow to develop into T and B cells. Thus, these infants have no immunity and usually die within the first few weeks of life.

**Acquired Defects in Immune Function**

*Overactivity and Autoimmunity*
One of the more important features of the immune system is discrimination between cells and tissues of the parent body ("self") and alien microorganisms ("nonself"). This ability is necessary to prevent immune responses from destroying the body they are supposed to defend. Autoimmunity is a disorder in which the immune system fails to recognize parts of the body as "self" and treats them as foreign, that is, it loses the ability to distinguish self from nonself. This can cause a variety of problems depending upon the extent of the immune responses and the part of the body involved. For example, autoimmune thyroiditis is a common organ-specific (only the thyroid gland is involved) autoimmune disease. Other autoimmune diseases, such as systemic lupus erythematosus (SLE) can affect many tissues throughout the body. The main problem in autoimmune diseases seems to be a defect in communication among the cells of the immune system. Either cells or antibody can cause damage, depending upon the tissue involved.

*Nutrition and Immunodeficiency*
Worldwide, the most common cause of acquired immune deficiency is malnutrition. It has been estimated that 500 million people, the majority of them children, suffer from malnutrition. Nutritional disorders are particularly common in underdeveloped countries, but have been shown to occur in all segments of the population, including hospitalized patients in the United States, Canada, and other industrialized countries. (The prevalence, severity, and types of infections found in malnourished persons are very similar to those seen in AIDS victims, that is, opportunistic infections by agents such as *P. carinii* and other viruses, bacteria, fungi, and protozoa.) Measles

and other common childhood viral infections have higher incidences of complications in children who are malnourished.

The most devastating effect of malnutrition is atrophy, or wasting, of the thymus gland. This has been recognized for many years. In fact, in 1845, a scientist wrote that "the thymus is a barometer of nutrition, and a very delicate one." The thymus reacts more rapidly than other organs to nutritional deficiencies and is the slowest to recover. The number of T cells in the circulation usually decreases with the loss of weight that occurs with malnutrition. Helper cells seem to be more affected than suppressor cells, particularly in children who have protein calorie malnutrition. Defects in nearly all T-cell functions have been detected. Along with effects on the thymus gland, it is suggested that changes in the number and function of immune cells are caused by decreases in the number of precursor cells and in survival time.

Overnutrition as well as undernutrition can cause immune deficiency. It has been shown that, in affluent societies, obesity (a form of malnutrition) is associated with increased respiratory infections and longer hospital stays following admission for routine procedures. In animal experiments, obesity has been found to be associated with greater susceptibility to viral and bacterial infections.

*Transplantation and Immunity*

Candidates for an organ transplant, e.g., a kidney or heart, from another person who is not an identical twin must have their immune systems suppressed so that the donor tissue will not be rejected. This is a form of acquired immune deficiency. Transplant patients are known to be especially susceptible to the same kinds of infections and cancers observed in AIDS patients. (The difference is that the cause of immune suppression in transplant patients is known.)

*Cancer and Immune Deficiency*

People who have cancers of certain types, especially of the lymph system, often become immunodeficient and develop serious infections. The toxic effects of drugs used to treat various types of cancers may also contribute to this immune deficiency.

*Other Causes of Immune Deficiency*

Almost any kind of stressful situation may lead to temporary immune suppression, due in part to increased amounts of corticosteroid hormones released during stress. Traumas such as burns, accidents, or surgery have been known to cause altered immune function. Pregnancy produces a temporary immunodeficient state, particularly during the last three months. It has been suggested that this temporary immunodeficiency is necessary to prevent the mother from rejecting the fetus as foreign tissue, but it also makes the mother susceptible to a number of viral infections. Immunodeficiency has also been associated with viral infections, especially CMV and Epstein-Barr virus (EBV), the cause of mononucleosis. Following infection, particularly with CMV, immune responses have been shown to be moderately decreased for up to a year. Finally, another cause of immunodeficiency is the intravenous (IV) use of drugs such as heroin. (The second largest group that develops AIDS is composed of IV-drug users.)

### THE IMMUNOLOGY OF AIDS

AIDS, as the name states, is a syndrome. This means that many different diseases and symptoms can combine and contribute to produce the overall state of ill health. This also means that the clinical picture of all AIDS patients is not identical. Since AIDS is a complex disease, it is not possible to combine all AIDS patients into one group and list exactly the associated changes in the immune system. However, AIDS patients do seem to fit into three general categories. Some AIDS patients have only Kaposi's sarcoma (KS) and no other symptoms of disease; another group has severe opportunistic infections such as *Pneumocystis carinii* pneumonia (PCP) or Candida (thrush); a third group has both KS and opportunistic infections. In general, patients in the third group tend to suffer the most severe changes in their immune systems, and patients with KS alone suffer the least severe changes.

In addition to AIDS, there is another immune-deficiency syndrome that occurs in homosexual men. This is the AIDS-Related Complex (ARC), and the number of ARC patients is much larger than the number of patients with overt AIDS. The manifestations of ARC include enlarged lymph nodes (glands) that persist over a period of months to years and may be associated with weight loss, fevers, night sweats, and a general malaise. It has been suggested by some physicians and researchers that ARC may be a pre-AIDS syndrome. This is disputed by others who think that ARC and AIDS are different. Immunologic changes are seen in patients with ARC, but they are not nearly as severe as those seen in patients with AIDS. Immune changes are also seen in healthy homosexual men.

AIDS is basically a disorder affecting the cellular, or T-cell, immune system, and exhibits the diseases associated with defective T-cell immunity, e.g., viral and fungal infections and cancers. In fact, the infections most often seen in AIDS patients and in renal transplant recipients are very similar. The largest percentage (70%) of people who develop AIDS are homosexual or bisexual men and, because of this, most immunologic studies have been done on blood and tissues from this population. (Later in this chapter, we will discuss some of the changes known to occur in other groups that get AIDS, e.g., hemophiliacs and IV-drug users.

Scientists have many different ways of testing immune function. First, cells or tissue can be removed from the body, and the numbers of different types of cells that are present can be counted. For example, lymphocytes can be separated from blood samples. As described earlier, there are many types of lymphocytes with different functions. Special antibodies, called monoclonal, have been developed which recognize particular structures on the surface of individual types of lymphocytes. When monoclonal antibodies are mixed with lymphocytes in a test tube, they recognize and attach to only those types of lymphocytes for which they are specific. This is a typical antigen-antibody reaction. By attaching other chemicals to the monoclonal antibodies, it becomes possible under a microscope to identify the lymphocytes with antibodies attached and to measure the percentage of lymphocytes of a particular type. The types of lymphocytes in bone marrow, lymph nodes, and other tissues of the body can similarly be measured. Using this technique, it is possible to measure the percentages of T helper, T suppressor, and B lymphocytes and NK cells.

In samples from AIDS patients it is not surprising that significant changes are seen in the numbers of T cells, since AIDS is a disorder of cellular immunity. The total number of T cells may or may not be decreased, but the percentage and absolute number of helper cells in the blood are significantly subnormal. This may sometimes, but not always, be accompanied by an increase in the number of suppressor cells. The result of the changes in helper and suppressor subpopulations is a decrease in what is called the $T_4$-to-$T_8$ ratio. The antigen on helper T cells recognized by monoclonal antibody is called the $T_4$ antigen, and the antigen specific for suppressor T cells and recognized by another monoclonal antibody is called the $T_8$ antigen. This is currently one of the most popular and easily performed tests for immune changes in patients with AIDS or suspected AIDS. However, this test is not specific for, or diagnostic of, AIDS, since other diseases such as viral infections also may be associated with changes in the $T_4$-to-$T_8$ ratio. The difference is that in patients with AIDS and ARC, NK cells, although they may not function normally (as will be discussed below), are normal or reduced in number.

Other tests can measure the various chemicals and substances associated with the immune system that are present in body fluids such as serum (obtained from blood). The quantities of different antibodies present, called the immunoglobulin levels, can thus be measured. The normal levels vary for people of different ages. In men with AIDS, and in some with ARC, immunoglobulin levels may be increased. IgG is the most common immunoglobulin to be increased, although IgA and IgM may be increased in certain instances. Some researchers have found that only IgA is increased in AIDS patients with KS. The increase in immunoglobulins raises the question as to how a deficient immune system can overreact and make larger rather than smaller amounts of antibody. The answer may be that the B cells make antibody nonspecifically without regulation by the defective T-cell system and cannot properly shut down antibody production. This can result in a continual pouring out of antibody that does not help defend against infectious agents.

Antibodies are not always protective and, in fact, can injure body tissues. If a large amount of antigen, such as virus, is present in the body, and if there are circulating antibodies to this antigen, then the antigen and antibody combine to form what are called immune complexes. Immune complexes can settle out in blood vessels or joints and cause severe damage with inflammation of the vessels and arthritis-like symptoms in the joints. Homosexual men with AIDS are infected with a variety of microorganisms, and many have been found to have high levels of circulating immune complexes. CMV may be one of the contributing factors in the development of KS, and it has been suggested by some scientists that immune complexes associated with CMV may deposit in blood vessels and lead to the high incidence of KS in AIDS patients.

Other immune complexes have been found with sperm components. Antibody to sperm and to parts of sperm have been measured in homosexual men, and high levels have been found in those with ARC or AIDS. This antibody is probably formed following the introduction of sperm during anal intercourse. Breaks, or lesions, in the rectum can facilitate entrance of these antigens into the blood. One type of antibody, specific to a chemical called asialo $GM_1$ present on the surface of sperm, may be especially important. Antibody to asialo $GM_1$ reacts with sperm, but can "cross-react" with helper T cells and NK cells. Perhaps antibody to asialo $GM_1$ contributes to the decrease in helper cells and the decrease in function of NK cells in men with AIDS.

Other substances that can be measured in fluids obtained from patients include lymphokines, secreted by cells of the immune system, which are used as one of the ways by which these cells communicate with one another. One type of lymphokine, called interleukin 2 (IL-2), is able to cause lymphocytes to divide and proliferate, thus increasing the number of lymphocytes reactive against specific antigens. This promotes a more effective immune response. In AIDS patients, IL-2 production may be defective, and it has been suggested that one way to treat these patients may be to enhance immune function by injecting IL-2. Another type of lymphokine, interferon, is produced during active viral infection. Interferon may act to increase the activity of NK cells, which in turn can destroy cells infected with virus. Interferon has been found circulating in the blood of some AIDS patients, indicating an ongoing viral infection.

Thymus hormones also can be measured in blood samples. There are several different types of thymic hormones, and a few laboratories have measured them in AIDS patients. The results of these studies were enigmatic; one type of thymus hormone was found to be increased and another was found to be decreased. A decrease in products of the thymus gland would not be surprising, especially in terminally ill AIDS victims, since the thymus gland becomes atrophied at this stage of disease.

In addition to measurements of numbers and amounts of cells and chemical substances in blood and tissue samples, many tests are available to measure the functional ability of cells. Virtually all such tests have revealed extreme abnormalities in AIDS patients. For example, when lymphocytes are placed in test tubes with chemicals called mitogens, or with cells from another person, the lymphocytes react by dividing. This is called a blastogenic or mitogenic response. In AIDS patients, this response is subnormal, implying that lymphocytes in the bodies of AIDS patients are defective and probably unable to divide normally after stimulation by antigen. Thus, the lymphocytes decrease not only in number but in their ability to mount an adequate immune response, which could lead to severe infections. Assays for NK-cell function also show abnormalities, some patients displaying virtually no NK activity. Since NK cells are important in controlling viral infections, defective activity (if it exists in the body as it does in the test tube) could lead to the persistent viral infections observed in many AIDS patients.

Some evaluations of immune function, such as skin tests, can be performed on the body (*in vivo*) rather than in a test tube (*in vitro*). Nearly all AIDS patients show decreased responses to skin tests with a variety of antigens, a further indication that their immune systems are unable to respond properly to the many agents they encounter. Their immune systems are said to have become anergic.

### Immune Changes in Other AIDS Groups

AIDS has also been reported in IV-drug users, Haitians, hemophiliacs, female sexual partners of AIDS victims, and children. With the exception of KS, which has been found only in homosexual men with AIDS, the spectrum of diseases in these groups is virtually identical to that in homosexual AIDS patients, as are the changes in the immune system: decreased $T_4$ helper lymphocytes, a decreased $T_4$-to-$T_8$ ratio, abnormal skin test responses, increased immunoglobulins, and defective NK-cell activity.

### SUMMARY

The immune system is a highly specialized, complex system that has developed to provide specific protection against foreign agents that enter the body. When the system malfunctions, debilitating diseases and death can result. The recently described acquired immune deficiency syndrome (AIDS), which occurs primarily in homosexual men, is a graphic example of what can happen when this system fails. AIDS is a disease of the immune system—all data indicate that the primary target for the agent(s) that causes AIDS is the immune system. The earliest detectable changes are in the numbers of circulating lymphocytes. These changes become worse, and the eventual effect is burnout of the immune system. The victim of AIDS then becomes totally unable to cope with foreign microorganisms and falls prey to these pathogens.

# 4    Signs and Symptoms
## of AIDS
### VICTOR GONG

AIDS is composed of many different diseases, and its signs and symptoms vary with the type and severity of the disease process. Many of these symptoms are common to other illnesses, such as everyday ailments like the common cold, and may be self-limiting and minor. None is specific to AIDS. You should be alerted, but not alarmed, if you have any one of these symptoms. However, if symptoms persist, consult your physician. Generally speaking, the following are the most common signs and symptoms of AIDS.

## PERSISTENT FEVERS OR NIGHT SWEATS

Fever is frequently the first sign that something is wrong with the body, usually an infection. The body's temperature is regulated by complex brain mechanisms. Normal body temperature is considered to be 98.6°F, taken orally, but can range from 97°F to 99.6°F. It also varies with age, body location, and time of day. You have a fever when your temperature is about 100.5°F in your mouth, above 101.5°F in your rectum, or above 99.5°F in your axilla (armpit). Chills and sweating may accompany the fevers. Drenching night sweats are characteristic of tuberculosis and frequently occur with AIDS. Many illnesses can cause fever, chills, or sweating, but persistence of these symptoms should prompt medical attention.

## SEVERE FATIGUE

Everyone goes through periods of tiredness. They may be due to a variety of stresses—overwork, emotional problems, dietary changes, etc. Profound fatigue lasting longer than several weeks and not easily attributable to such stresses, or to psychiatric or medication effects, may be an early signal of a serious illness.

## WEIGHT LOSS

An unexplained weight loss of 10 or more pounds, or greater than 10% of one's body weight, during a period of less than 2 months may indicate illness. Loss of appetite often accompanies the weight loss. These symptoms may be due to many causes, such as exercise, dieting, emotional or psychological problems, endocrine disorders, infections, and cancers, as well as AIDS, AIDS-related complex, or the lymphadenopathy syndrome. If your appetite does not return and weight loss persists with no obvious cause, seek medical attention.

## SWOLLEN GLANDS (LYMPHADENOPATHY)

Lymph nodes, located strategically throughout the body (in the neck, groin, armpits, etc.), are part of the body's defense against infection. They may become swollen due to infection, malignancies, or reactions to drugs, and simply indicate an active immune system at work. Glands of the groin and neck regions commonly become enlarged, sometimes without obvious cause. Viral (e.g., the flu or mononucleosis) and bacterial (e.g., tuberculosis) infections can cause lymph node enlargement, sometimes for weeks. The condition termed lymphadenopathy—enlarged, hard, sometimes painful nodes in at least two parts of the body (excluding the groin) for more than 3 months—may indicate AIDS or a prodromal AIDS condition called the lymphadenopathy syndrome.

## ORAL THRUSH

Oral thrush is an infection of the tongue and mouth caused by a yeast, *Candida albicans*. Candida is normally present in the mouth

and gastrointestinal tract, but causes serious trouble only during debilitating illness, malnutrition, or the taking of antibiotics that suppress the normal balance of microorganisms and allow overgrowth of
the fungus. Thrush is a persistent, creamy-white, curdlike patch that
coats the tongue, surrounding throat, and esophagus (the food pipe
that connects the throat to the stomach). It may be painful and cause
difficulty in swallowing, but rarely involves other internal organs.

## PERSISTENT DIARRHEA

Diarrhea is frequent and loose bowel movements, usually signifying
an attempt by the body to rid itself of an irritant or harmful substance. It may be due to toxins, infections, cancers, diet, emotional
stress, or a host of other causes. Persistent diarrhea (longer than one
week) is not normal and may lead to severe dehydration and loss of
essential body salts.

## COUGHING AND/OR SHORTNESS OF BREATH

An unusual pneumonia, such as *Pneumocystis carinii* pneumonia,
often appears with AIDS. It may begin as a cough, a normal clearing
action of the lung in which a reflex triggered by irritation of the airways expels debris, pus, and pathogens. The cough may produce
phlegm or be dry. In AIDS, however, the cough may persist for
weeks and progress to shortness of breath, indicating more severe
damage to the respiratory system. A prolonged cough accompanied
by fevers, chills, tightness in the chest, and increased respiratory and
pulse rates is an early warning of pneumonia. Shortness of breath not
associated with heavy exertion, excitement, or a blocked nasal condition also warrants medical attention.

## SKIN RASHES AND SPOTS

Lumps, bumps, and rashes on the skin always cause concern and
create anxieties about possible cancer. In AIDS, the fear of Kaposi's
sarcoma (KS) is especially prevalent. The lesions of KS vary. They
are painless and non-itching, range in size from an insect bite to large
nodules or plaques, are colored brown, blue, or purple, and may be

found anywhere on the skin. Other skin lesions may develop inside the nose, mouth, or anus as a consequence of recurrent herpes ulcers of various malignancies.

## BRUISING OR BLEEDING

Easy bruising and bleeding occur in some AIDS patients. Cuts may take longer to clot, mucous membranes may bleed without prior trauma, and even minor injuries may result in bruising. An uncommon blood disorder, autoimmune thrombocytopenia purpura (ATP), has been noted in gay men at the same times and places as the AIDS epidemic, suggesting a causal relationship. In ATP, a defective immune system makes antibodies to destroy platelets, blood elements necessary for normal clotting. Any unusual bruising or bleeding should be reported to a physician.

## NEUROLOGICAL PROBLEMS

A great variety of nervous system diseases and disorders appears in AIDS patients. These complaints may include headaches, stiff neck, pain, numbness, or weakness of the extremities, and even psychiatric symptoms such as depression, delusions, hallucinations, and paranoia. Most common in one study of AIDS patients were headache and fatigue. The apparent benignity of some neurological complaints may lead the unsuspecting patient and physician astray. The pathology in these patients is diverse, ranging from brain infections (meningitis and encephalitis) or brain tumors and lymphomas to brain hemorrhages. Anyone with neurologic disease who also belongs to one of the risk groups for AIDS should be given an extensive neurological evaluation, which may include CAT scans (cross-sectional x-rays) of the head, spinal taps, open brain biopsy, and other laboratory tests. Some of these conditions are treatable if diagnosed early enough.

# 5     The Infections of AIDS

Opportunistic infections are well known in patients with either congenital or acquired immunodeficiency. There are many individuals who are born with absent or weakened immune systems and so are prone to opportunistic infections. Cancer patients and those treated with chemotherapy or radiation are also at risk. More recently, patients with organ transplantation who have to be treated with drugs to prevent rejection of the newly acquired organs are also candidates for serious opportunistic infections. In AIDS, opportunistic infections are associated with a defective cell-mediated immunity and include many varieties of bacteria, fungi, viruses and parasites. These diseases are regarded as "markers" for the underlying AIDS. Three classes of infections—viral, parasitic, and bacterial and fungal— their characteristics, spectrum of illnesses, and clinical course are described in the following chapter.

## A.   Viral Infections
### HELEN L. LIPSCOMB

Viral infections are probably the most common illnesses of both man and animals. They range in severity from causing no symptoms to inducing debilitation or death. Certain viruses are also oncogenic, i.e., cancer-causing.

Viral infections are especially important in the consideration of the acquired immune deficiency syndrome (AIDS). Indeed, AIDS may be a direct result of infection by a new virus that specifically attacks the immune system. Although the "new virus" has not yet been conclusively verified, it is known that AIDS is a disease of the immune system, especially the T-cell immune system. People with defective T-cell immunity are particularly susceptible to infections by viruses, and AIDS victims do fall prey to repeated viral infections.

Also important is the connection between viruses and cancers. It is known that many of the viruses that plague AIDS patients have also been linked to the types of cancers AIDS patients develop. This section of the chapter will define what a virus is, describe how the body normally defends itself against viral infections, and discuss the viral infections most often associated with AIDS.

## WHAT IS A VIRUS?

Virus is a term for a group of extremely small microorganisms that cannot live or reproduce outside of living cells. They must enter a host cell in order to use much of the cell's biosynthetic machinery for their own replication. This pirating of the cell by the virus causes the initial symptoms of viral infections. Once a virus enters a cell, it instructs that cell to make more virus which then leaves to infect other cells. This process continues until the infection is either recognized and halted by the host's immune system or the infection becomes overwhelming and causes death.

Certain viruses, especially of the herpes family, can remain inactive within the host cell for long periods without causing problems. They remain integrated with the cell's genetic material (DNA) until triggered to begin replication, a property called *viral latency*. The previously dormant virus is said to be *reactivated*. For example, a first infection with herpesvirus type I (oral herpes) is often asymptomatic. After the initial infection, the virus lives in nerve cells of the face from which it may be reactivated at intervals and cause characteristic fever blisters. The exact triggers of reactivation are not known, but associated factors may include exposure to ultraviolet light, fever, the presence of other infections, and immunodeficiency.

When a virus enters a cell and begins to reproduce, the immediate damage may vary from none to total destruction of the cell. In many viral infections, reproduction by undamaged cells quickly replaces the destroyed cells. However, destruction of epithelial surfaces (linings) of the respiratory tract, common in some viral respiratory infections such as influenza, compromises normal defense mechanisms and makes the host more susceptible to infection by invading bacteria. This is called secondary bacterial infection. Some cells, especially of nerves, are not able to reproduce and are thus not replaced after infection by a virus. The most vivid example of this is polio in which viral replication destroys the nerve cells (motoneurons) that control muscle movement and produces paralysis.

## HOW DOES THE BODY DEFEND AGAINST VIRAL INFECTIONS?

Depending upon the severity of the infection, the body's main defenses against viral infections are inflammation, antibody formation, interferon production, and cellular immunity.

### Inflammation

Inflammation in blood vessels and adjacent tissues is a typical response to any type of infection. The ultimate purpose of inflammation is to remove the offending agent(s) and to repair and heal injured tissue. Signs include redness, heat, swelling, and pain. Redness and heat are due to locally increased fluid and leakage of cells out of the blood vessels. Pain is caused by stimulation of nerve endings due to pressure in the area.

### Antibodies

Many different antibodies are formed in response to viral infections. They may be thought of as the "footprints" of a virus and tell us what type of virus we are dealing with and how long ago it was there. The antibodies include three main classes: IgM, IgA, and IgG.

As in other infections, virus-specific IgM is produced early in the disease and is a good indicator of current or recent infection. IgA, or secretory, antibodies are an important part of the immune response to viral infections. Their presence in nasal passages and airways and in intestinal secretions defends against further infection by respiratory or intestinal viruses. IgG antibodies indicate past infection and a successful defense against the infecting virus.

### Interferon

Interferon proteins are produced by cells, especially of the macrophage system, in response to viral infection and may be partly responsible for ending an infection. They are not antibodies and are specific for the host species in which they are produced rather than for the agent that induced their formation. (Antibodies are specific for the invading agent.) Thus, human infections must be treated with interferon produced by human cells. Interferon interferes with viral synthesis and thus inhibits the spread of the infection.

### Cellular Immunity

Cellular, or T-cell, immunity also helps to end viral infections. T cells have a cytotoxic (cell-damaging) effect that destroys virus-infected cells. They also attract macrophages, which are responsible for phagocytosis (engulfing) and destruction of viral particles and cell debris. A special type of T cell, called a memory T cell, also is produced during an immune response. Memory T cells persist in the body for a long time and "remember" a particular type of virus. Because of these cells, later exposure to the "remembered" viruses evokes a speedier immune response and, if the immune system is normal, quick destruction of the invading virus. Another type of immune cell, called the natural killer (NK) cell, is the body's first line of defense against virus-infected cells and certain types of tumor cells.

### VIRAL INFECTIONS OF AIDS PATIENTS

AIDS victims are particularly susceptible to infection with herpesviruses. These include herpes simplex types I and II, varicella-zoster (chickenpox-shingles), cytomegalovirus (CMV), and Epstein-Barr virus (EBV). Herpesviruses have a unique relationship to humans in that they are able to combine with the genetic material, DNA, of certain cells of a human host and to remain latent for long periods, possibly for the life of the host. As mentioned earlier, the factors that control latency and reactivation are not well understood. The many recurrences of herpes simplex or varicella-zoster infections seen in otherwise healthy people are commonly associated with immunodeficiency.

### Cytomegaloviruses

CMV is a particular group of host-specific herpesviruses that infects man and other animals. Many specifically affect salivary glands and cause enlargement of cells in various organs of the body. CMV can infect in three ways: (1) in the developing fetus (congenital), (2) as a primary infection in nonimmune persons, and (3) by reactivation of latent infection in immunosuppressed patients.

Congenital CMV disease follows infection of a nonimmune mother during the early months of pregnancy. The effects on the fetus are variable, but stillbirth or neonatal death can occur. Some of the infants who survive may exhibit no evidence of having been exposed to the disease; others suffer severe damage of the central nervous system, liver, lungs, kidneys, and other tissues.

Primary infection in nonimmune persons is normally mild and mainly in children and young adults. It is transmitted by droplet infection or contact with the secretions of congenitally infected infants. Clinical symptoms are fever, fatigue, sore throat, and enlarged lymph glands. In fact, primary CMV infection resembles mononucleosis (the virus that usually causes mononucleosis is EBV, discussed below).

Latent CMV infections may be reactivated in immunosuppressed persons. Because of this, it is not surprising that virtually all patients with AIDS have antibody to CMV, and a large percentage of homosexual men with AIDS actually excrete the virus in saliva and semen. It has been found that people with normal immune systems, experiencing CMV infection for the first time, display an immunosuppression that may last for weeks or months. Thus, it is possible that, in AIDS patients, reactivated and persistent CMV infections add to and compound the immunosuppression and increase the severity of the disease. CMV may also play a part in the development of Kaposi's sarcoma, common in AIDS patients. It has been isolated in Kaposi's lesions, and some think CMV may be oncogenic (cancer-causing). No effective methods are known for the prevention or treatment of CMV infections.

**Epstein-Barr Virus**

EBV, another member of the herpesvirus family, causes infectious mononucleosis ("mono," or the "kissing disease"). It has also been associated with two types of cancers: Burkitt's lymphoma and nasopharyngeal carcinoma. EBV is unique among viruses in that it infects cells of the immune system—B cells—responsible for making antibody. B cells have specific receptors for EBV. The virus attaches to the receptors and enters the cells where it reproduces. Like the CMV mono-like disease, EBV-induced mono is usually a mild disease of children and young adults. However, EBV also is able to remain latent and to become subsequently reactivated. Almost all homosexual men with AIDS have antibodies to EBV, compared to an 85–95% incidence in healthy adults. AIDS patients also suffer significant reactivation of EBV infections, as indicated by the types of antibodies found, and tend to develop lymphomas of B cells (resembling Burkitt's lymphoma) for which it has been suggested that EBV may be at least partly responsible.

**Herpes Simplex Virus**

The two main types of herpes simplex virus (HSV) infections are caused by HSV type I (*herpes labialis*—fever blister, cold sore) and HSV type II (genital, or venereal, herpes). As with the other types of herpesviruses, these two are notorious for their ability to remain latent and to become periodically reactivated. Cold sores are the most common HSV type I infection, and it has been estimated that 20–40% of the population of the United States have recurrent infections with this virus. The characteristic lesions are fluid-filled pustules at the edges of the lips containing viral particles capable of infecting others.

HSV type II is transmitted as a venereal infection and has been associated with cervical cancer. With genital herpes, the primary infection may be asymptomatic, and then, some time later, the characteristic lesions may appear on the penis of males or in the cervix, vagina, and anal areas of females. However, lesions sometimes appear soon after the first contact with the virus. One of the most serious consequences of HSV II is neonatal herpes infection of babies during childbirth. Premature newborns and infants with debilitating diseases or immunodeficiency are particularly vulnerable. The disease ranges from a mild illness to a fulminating systemic infection with enlarged lymph glands and necrotic lesions throughout the body. The fatality rate in severe cases is very high, and infants who survive often have permanent brain damage.

HSV type II is extremely common in AIDS patients. It is seen in homosexual men, most commonly as a recurrent ulcer around the anus. Because AIDS patients are immunosuppressed, episodes of viral reactivation are more numerous. Two of the common types of cancers that occur in AIDS patients may be associated with HSV: squamous cell carcinoma of the tongue with HSV type I, and carcinoma of the rectum with HSV type II.

### Varicella-Zoster Virus

Chickenpox (varicella) is a primary infection of a nonimmune host by a varicella-zoster virus (VZV). It is contracted by inhalation of virus-infected droplets. The virus migrates from the respiratory tract to the lymphatic system and spreads to the lymph glands. It replicates there and enters the bloodstream, to be carried to the skin and mucous membranes where it produces characteristic blisters.

In children, chickenpox is a mild illness characterized by fever, a rash (particularly on the trunk), and often blisters in the mouth. Complications are rare in children, but in adults the disease is more severe and the risk of complications, such as pneumonia, higher.

### Shingles (Zoster)

Shingles (herpes zoster) is caused by reactivation of VZV, thought to remain latent in nerve cells after an attack of chickenpox. As with other herpesviruses, reactivation is more likely in immunocompromised individuals. Thus, shingles is common in AIDS patients, and some cases have been especially severe.

### Hepatitis

Hepatitis simply means inflammation of the liver. Many different viruses can infect and damage the liver, e.g., herpesvirus hominis, CMV, EBV, coxsackieviruses, and certain insect-carried viruses (arboviruses) found in tropical countries. Usually, however, so-called viral hepatitis is the term used for liver disease caused by hepatitis A or B viruses (HAV or HBV). Hepatitis caused by the other agents is called non-A non-B hepatitis.

Hepatitis A-like illness was described by Hippocrates 2000 years ago. Sporadic cases and epidemics have been reported over the centuries, and to this day hepatitis remains a common disease. Type A hepatitis has an incubation period of about 2 to 6 weeks (for hepatitis B the period averages 2 to 6 months, but is sometimes much shorter). As the virus disappears from the stool, antibody levels rise quickly in the blood and remain detectable for at least 10 years. This gives long-lasting immunity against reinfection.

Type A hepatitis is usually transmitted from person to person by the fecal-oral route. It may also be spread by contaminated food, water, and shellfish. Infection is most common in children, lower socioeconomic groups, and rural rather than urban dwellers. During active infection, virus is present in the blood for only a short time and in small amounts. Because of this, transmission by blood transfusion is uncommon, in contrast to non-A non-B hepatitis and hepatitis B.

Hepatitis B differs from hepatitis A in many ways, including viral structure, method of transmission, length of incubation period, severity of infection, and the existence of a chronic hepatitis B carrier state. The sources of HBV infection are chronic carriers of the virus and patients with acute hepatitis B. In both sources, virus particles may be found in blood and other body secretions. A carrier state develops in 5% to 10% of infected persons, and it has been estimated that there are 120 million carriers throughout the world. The carrier rate varies with geographic location: in the United States, it is about 0.1% of the population, as compared to more than 15% in some tropical areas.

HBV is transmitted mainly by inoculation. The transfusion of blood and blood products obtained from infected donors, the use of contaminated syringes and needles by drug abusers, and the use of contaminated surgical equipment are frequent modes of infection. A high carrier rate is found among transplant recipients, patients who have received multiple blood transfusions, and people with immuno deficiency disorders. A tiny drop of infected blood can transmit the virus, and even shared toothbrushes and razor blades are potential instruments of inoculation. In fact, injection is not the only route of infection; the virus has been found in urine, saliva, semen, menstrual blood, and other body fluids and secretions. With such widespread contamination of body fluids, oral, sexual, or intimate physical contact of any kind can result in HBV transmission.

The incubation period for hepatitis B ranges from 6 to 180 days, depending upon how much virus was injected. The pathological effects of HAV and HBV on the liver are virtually identical. Infection by either virus causes structural and functional changes in the liver ranging from insignificant to severe and irreversible.

Despite similarities in the pathologic changes produced in the liver, there are important differences between the outcomes of HAV and HBV diseases. For HAV, complete recovery within a few weeks is the rule, and complications are rare. For HBV, a few patients rapidly develop fatal necrosis of the liver; about 10% develop a continuing chronic infection that sometimes causes symptoms and sometimes does not. Many patients who develop chronic HBV infections do so without going through a phase of overt acute hepatitis.

AIDS patients show evidence of infection with both HAV and HBV. The incidence of antibodies to and infection with HAV is similar to that seen in the general population. In contrast, the carrier rate for HBV is extremely high in AIDS patients and in homosexual men with pre-AIDS-like syndromes. Of importance to groups of patients at risk for developing AIDS is the recent development and release of an anti-HBV vaccine produced from the pooled plasma of donors who test positive for hepatitis antigen. There was initial concern that the agent responsible for causing AIDS might be transmitted with the anti-HBV vaccine, but this has not happened. Several thousand volunteer health-care workers received the vaccine between 1975 and 1983, and none developed AIDS. Since the vaccine was placed on the market in July 1982, over 200,000 persons have received it and no cases of AIDS have been reported outside of high-risk groups.

**Adenovirus**

Adenoviruses cause respiratory tract infections that range in severity from the common cold to viral pneumonia. They can also cause eye infections, which frequently accompany adenoviral respiratory tract diseases. These infections are generally mild and produce few complications. However, in patients who are immunosuppressed, e.g., due to AIDS or treatment for an organ transplant, the adenovirus can cause severe disturbances and spread throughout the body. There is no successful treatment for infections by this virus.

**Human T-cell Leukemia Viruses**

Retroviruses were discovered in animals about 20 years ago. They are known to cause cancers, especially leukemias, in mice, cats, monkeys, and birds. Recently, human-specific retroviruses have been isolated. In Japan and certain areas of the Caribbean, a human T-cell leukemia virus (HTLV-I), a retrovirus, is associated with T-cell malignancies, and a large percentage of people in areas where these malignancies are endemic have antibodies to this virus. Since HTLV-1 infects primarily T-helper lymphocytes, some initially believed that this was the cause of AIDS. However, two other retroviruses, which may prove to be identical to each other, have also been found in AIDS patients. The first, lymphadenopathy virus (LAV) was isolated at the Pasteur Institute in France, and the second, HTLV-III, was isolated in the United States. Antibodies to these viruses have been found in AIDS and pre-AIDS patients, and the viruses themselves have been isolated from a number of AIDS victims. Whether HTLV-III/LAV cause(s) AIDS or is just another opportunistic infection in severely compromised AIDS victims remains to be determined.

## SUMMARY

There is no doubt that viruses are extremely important in the etiology of AIDS. Depending upon the type of virus, consequences can be immune depression, overwhelming opportunistic infection, and cancers of various types. It is not known whether viruses alone are sufficient to produce AIDS, or whether a single agent acts as a trigger to initiate the irreversible immune depression characteristic of AIDS.

# B.   Parasitic Infections
## NIRMAL K. FERNANDO AND PETER HO

### *PNEUMOCYSTIS CARINII*

Most AIDS patients will be diagnosed as having *Pneumocystis carinii* pneumonia (PCP) when first seen by a physician; PCP is also the leading cause of AIDS deaths. PCP is an opportunistic infection whose importance has increased over the past decade, due, in part, to the advent of effective chemotherapy for cancer patients.

In the United States, PCP was not reported until 1956, when it was first noted in children with congenital immune defects. The mode of transmission and natural habitat of *Pneumocystis carinii*, the parasite microorganism that causes PCP, remain largely unknown. It has been found in the lungs of animals and of normal, healthy humans, and autopsy studies have occasionally shown the organisms in the lungs of patients who had no immune defect. However, no documented cases of PCP have been reported in adults with intact immune systems.

The severity of PCP in AIDS patients may obscure the fact that its ability to flourish is due to a weakened immune system rather than to the infectiousness of the parasite. The parasite multiplies and fills the air spaces in the lungs, provoking an intense inflammatory response and the clinical manifestation of pneumonia.

#### Clinical Manifestations of PCP

Most AIDS patients have already been ill for some time before they get PCP. Weight loss, low grade fever, diarrhea, and unexplained lymph node enlargement often precede pulmonary involvement, although fever and cough are the first complaints. Gradually, the cough becomes worse and shortness of breath develops, especially with physical exertion. Interestingly, a stethoscope often reveals no abnormal sounds in the lungs, even though chest x-rays may show pneumonia on both sides. A small percentage of AIDs patients with PCP have a more rapid and severe onset with high fever, rapidly progressive shortness of breath, and profuse sweating. The pneumonia prevents the transport of oxygen from inhaled air into the blood, lowering blood oxygen to dangerous levels. The following is a typical PCP case:

A 41-year-old intravenous-drug abuser noticed weakness, easy fatigability, and a nonproductive cough in July 1983. He attributed this to a viral infection and was able to continue his activities, although he became short-winded when he jogged. His physician prescribed an antibiotic. The shortness of breath got worse and he was hospitalized in September 1983. By then he had a fever, night sweats, and a persistent cough. He was initially treated for bacterial pneumonia, and his symptoms improved slightly over the next 2 weeks. However, he then became markedly short of breath and breathed very rapidly. He deteriorated quickly and, even with aggressive therapy, died 5 days later.

**Diagnosis**

No characteristic symptoms are definitive for PCP. Blood gas usually shows decreased oxygen, especially after exercise. Chest x-rays are often normal at first but, as the disease advances, bilateral infiltrate (haziness on the x-ray) is the most common pattern. Interestingly, in the early stages, when the chest x-ray is normal, a simultaneous gallium scan usually shows active uptake in the lungs. (Gallium is a metallic element preferentially taken up by certain inflammatory cells in the body.) The definitive diagnosis of PCP requires the identification of the organism in samples taken from the lung.

Lung tissue is usually obtained directly by biopsy using a flexible bronchoscope. If this fails to decide the diagnosis, open-lung biopsy is the final step. In bronchoscopy, which is less invasive than open-lung biopsy, a small tube is passed down the trachea (windpipe) and into the lung. In an open-lung biopsy, a small incision is made on the chest wall, one or two small segments of ribs are cut away, and lung tissue is obtained through the incision.

**Therapy**

Specific antibiotics for PCP are highly effective but the underlying immunosuppression usually results in frequent relapses. Clotrimoxazole, a combination of sulfamethoxazole and trimethoprim antibiotics in a fixed ratio and commonly used to treat urinary tract infections, is also used for PCP but in much larger doses and for longer periods. The other antibiotic most frequently used for PCP is pentamidine, available only from the Centers for Disease Control, a government agency. Clotrimoxazole causes rashes more often in AIDS patients than in the general population.

In the United States, most physicians initially treat PCP with intravenous trimethoprim/sulfamethoxazole (Bactrim or Septra) since it is believed to be the less toxic of the two drugs. If the patient does not improve, pentamidine is either added to the Bactrim or substituted for it. The complete blood count and kidney and liver functions must be carefully monitored when these drugs are administered because of their known adverse effects on bone marrow (where blood cells are made) and on the kidneys and liver. Another serious, but relatively uncommon, side effect is severe hypoglycemia (low blood sugar). Also, because pentamidine given intravenously may cause an irregular heart rhythm, it is most often injected into muscle tissue. Both pentamidine and Bactrim have been reported to cause a mild and transient inflammation of the nerves (peripheral neuritis).

A major problem for AIDS patients is that both relapse and reinfection are common due to continued immunosuppression. It is unfortunate that the immunologic impairment in AIDS is not reversible, since correction of the immunosuppression would lead to spontaneous recovery from the infection. Taking medications prophylactically to prevent infections has been proposed and even practiced by some authorities, but judgment of the effectiveness of prophylaxis awaits further clinical studies.


## TOXOPLASMOSIS

*Toxoplasma gondii*, like *Pneumocystis carinii*, is a parasite that lives in a latent, asymptomatic state in many healthy people. It is distributed worldwide and affects virtually all mammalian species. Humans may acquire the organism through contaminated food, blood transfusions, or organ transplantation, and *in utero* (transmitted to the unborn fetus via the placenta). Drinking contaminated water, or eating undercooked meat, such as pork, beef, or veal, or food contaminated by cat feces, may lead to infection. Pet cats are a well-known source of *T. gondii* infection.

## Clinical Manifestations

In AIDS, this asymptomatic infection involves all organs of the body, with especially devastating effects on the brain (encephalitis) that have been particularly common in Haitians who have contracted AIDS. Brain symptoms include confusion, headache, weakness, dizziness, seizures, and other characteristics resembling a stroke. This type of symptom complex mimics that of a brain tumor. The patient is very sick and often deteriorates rapidly to death.

Pneumonia can also occur as the organism attacks the lungs. Thus cough, fever, shortness of breath, and an abnormal chest x-ray are helpful clues to diagnosis.

Another organ commonly affected in immunosuppressed patients is the heart muscle. Heart infection is called myocarditis (from the Latin words for muscle and heart). Changes in heart rate and rhythm, observed in an electrocardiogram, together with a general physical examination establish this serious diagnosis. Myocarditis can result in heart failure and, if compounded with pneumonia, may be life-threatening.

## Diagnosis

A definite diagnosis of *T. gondii* infection requires a biopsy of the suspected organ. The organism can then be identified by a pathologist after the tissue sample is properly processed and examined. Blood tests are usually helpful, but often show deceptively normal responses in AIDS patients. A brain scan and a CAT scan (special cross-sectional x-ray) of the head may be helpful, but are not definitive.

## Therapy

Treatment consists of general supportive measures directed at the particular organ involved. For example, if the patient has a pneumonia, the antibiotic combination of sulfadiazine and pyrimethamine is given. Repetitive courses of medication are often necessary, since complete cure is never achieved. However, this antibiotic has a dangerous side effect on blood-cell production in the bone marrow so that in AIDS, when the blood count is invariably abnormal, the addition of this drug complication would be detrimental. This again indicates that the diseases to which AIDS patients are subject are very dangerous, and that some of the medications used to combat them can lead to serious complications.

## AMEBIASIS AND GIARDIASIS

For over a decade before the outbreak of AIDS, physicians found in homosexuals a large number of intestinal parasites once thought to be exclusively in the domain of tropical diseases. The associated enteric infections were named the "gay bowel syndrome," and included common venereal diseases such as gonorrhea and syphilis as well as others less generally considered venereal, for example, shigellosis, amebiasis, and giardiasis. Amebiasis and giardiasis are among the most common diarrheal diseases in AIDS. They are caused by intestinal parasites that can exist in a latent, asymptomatic state or create severe disturbances. The usual mode of transmission of the organisms is through contaminated food or drink. However, in homosexuals the anal-oral route is prevalent due to the pattern of sexual practices.

### Amebiasis

Amebiasis is caused by *Entameba histolytica* and is characterized by lower abdominal cramps, fever, and bloody diarrhea. Since only about 10% of patients become symptomatic, the infection is largely spread by healthy "carriers." In the United States in general the prevalence is 3% to 4%, but in the homsexual population of New York City the figure is closer to 40%. The organism is found in soil and water, but man is the principal host and source of infection.

Diagnosis is made by identifying the organism in the stool or in material scraped from the inner lining of the lower bowel. Identifying parasites in the stool requires special experience and training, since these infections are relatively uncommon in the United States.

*E. histolytica* may spread to the liver but rarely to other organs. In nonbowel amebiasis, blood tests are most commonly used for diagnosis although the organism can sometimes be observed in pus collected from the abscess. Diagnosis of amebiasis is not a major problem in AIDS.

A drug called metronidazole (Flagyl) has been used successfully to treat amebiasis, but, depending on the site of infections, other medications may be necessary.

### Giardiasis

Giardiasis is the most common waterborne, epidemic diarrheal illness in the United States. It is caused by *Giardia lamblia*, a protozoan of worldwide distribution. Campers, particularly in the Rocky Mountains, have been infected after drinking untreated water from mountain streams, but the infection has also been found all over the country. Asymptomatic carriers can transmit the nonvegetative, or cyst, form of the organism. The organism resides in the upper part of the small intestine.

Symptoms vary, but typically include an explosive, watery, foul-smelling diarrhea, abdominal distention, and flatulence. Nausea, vomiting, fever, and blood in the stools are uncommon, but belching is frequent. Some patients present with chronic intermittent diarrhea and weight loss.

Treatment is with quinacrine, considered the drug of choice, or with metronidazole (Flagyl). Quinacrine may induce abdominal pains, headaches, and a yellow discoloration of the skin and urine. Drinking alcohol during medication with quinacrine produces a violent reaction characterized by nausea, vomiting, and abdominal pain.

## CRYPTOSPORIDIOSIS

Cryptosporidium is a tiny protozoan parasite that causes cryptosporidiosis, diarrhea in animals, especially calves. Mild diarrhea can afflict infected humans, but human infection usually resolves itself spontaneously. Often, the organism is not recognized as the cause of diarrhea because the illness is self-limiting and stools may not have been examined specifically for cryptosporidium. In AIDS, however, cryptosporidiosis is a devastating infection characterized by unrelenting, voluminous, watery diarrhea progressing to dehydration, loss of important body salts, and malnutrition. The clinical picture is similar to that of cholera in which the patient can die from the complications of dehydration and malnutrition. With severe dehydration, the blood pressure drops, leading to a state of shock.

There is no effective therapy or drug at present to eradicate this parasite, although many have been tried. Treatment is directed at maintaining fluid and nutritional balance by supportive measures such as intravenous infusions. Since there is no cure, diarrhea recurs intermittently.

## SUMMARY

AIDS patients are susceptible to a variety of parasitic infections. Most common is PCP, which is also the primary cause of AIDS deaths. The other infections are primarily diarrheal, and many are quite common. While they may cause extreme discomfort in otherwise healthy individuals, they rarely result in serious illness. AIDS patients, however, may present with the infection for prolonged periods and become dangerously malnourished. Malnutrition may sometimes become severe enough to be fatal.

---

# C.   Bacterial and Fungal Infections

## JOHN W. SENSAKOVIC, EDWARD JOHNSON, AND VICTOR GONG

We are constantly surrounded by many different types of microorganisms, including bacteria and fungi. Most prominent are bacteria, single-celled organisms barely visible under the microscope but capable of both harm and benefit to man. The air we breathe and the food we eat, no matter how carefully prepared, are tainted with bacteria and sometimes cause serious illness.

Our bodies are host to many organisms. The mouth harbors streptococci, pneumococci, and other organisms that cause penumonia, ear and throat infections, etc. The bowel contains millions of bacteria, some of which have such beneficial functions as the synthesis of vitamins, while others can cause serious disease. The delicate balance between bacterial infections and a healthy coexistence is disrupted in AIDS. Seemingly benign bacteria can become fatal enemies. This chapter will describe the most common bacterial and fungal infections seen in AIDS, but any number of other infectious microbes can potentially complicate the existence of AIDS victims.

## BACTERIAL INFECTIONS

### Tuberculosis

Tuberculosis, almost forgotten in this modern era of antibiotics, has been recorded since ancient times as a feared and dangerous disease. The name derives from the Latin word *tuberculum*, or lump, describing the small masses caused by *Mycobacterium tuberculosis*, the tubercle bacillus. This microbe is most often spread by infected sputum droplets, but may also appear in unpasteurized dairy products. Although the microbe can attack virtually any organ of the body, the lung is usually the site of infestation (called pulmonary tuberculosis).

Symptoms vary. Early in the disease, patients may have no symptoms, although some experience fatigue, low grade fevers, loss of appetite, and weight loss. As the disease progresses, a cough, purulent (sometimes bloody) sputum, night sweats, chest pains, and shortness of breath occur. Eventually, if the disease is untreated, the tubercle bacillus may spread to other organs, and the victim becomes emaciated and dies.

Diagnosis is made by clinical examination, simple skin tests, chest x-rays, and isolation of the organism, usually from the sputum. Many individuals have probably been exposed to the bacillus yet most have not contracted any active disease. Exposed individuals develop antibodies to the bacillus, an important defense mechanism by which the body fights off future invasions by the bacteria. Scientists have developed special skin tests to detect those who have either been exposed to tuberculosis or have an active infection. An extract of the bacteria is injected just beneath the skin, and previously exposed or currently infected subjects normally develop a red lump in the area of injection. However, no skin induration develops in AIDS patients, regardless of the presence of disease, because their impaired immunity prevents the development of antibodies necessary for a positive skin test. Chest x-rays will show areas of scarring or infiltrates in the lung, and cultures of sputum from AIDS patients will grow the tuberculosis bacteria.

While tuberculosis is not considered an opportunistic infection, and many patients other than those with AIDS may acquire the disease, it quite often accompanies AIDS. The infection is even more fulminant and difficult to eradicate in these patients than in those with intact immunity.

The treatment of tuberculosis was futile prior to the advent of potent antibiotics. The drugs used consist of a combination including isoniazid, rifampin, ethambutol, and streptomycin because the bacillus may develop resistance if only a single antituberculosis drug is used. Treatment must be continued for at least a year in usual tuberculosis cases.

### Atypical Tuberculosis

The term tuberculosis traditionally refers to infections with the bacterium, *M. tuberculosis*. However, in recent years, modern microbiological techniques have identified other forms of tuberculosis in man, named "atypical mycobacterial infections."

In October 1982, the first cluster of atypical mycobacterial infections was reported in New York City among homosexuals and intravenous-drug abusers. The particular infections that have been implicated are designated *Mycobacterium avium-intracellulare* (MAI), which includes *M. avium* and *M. intracellulare*. These pathogens are common in our environment, e.g., in soil, water, house dust, and even in our mouths. Except in high-risk groups, they rarely cause disease in man.

MAI infections, although not as virulent or destructive as typical tuberculosis, produce a disease that is clinically indistinguishable from it. The most common location of the disease is the lung; but, as in tuberculosis, any organ may be involved. This atypical pulmonary infection generally occurred in middle-aged men with immunosuppressive disorders and was usually chronic and slowly progressive, rarely disseminating to other organs. Dissemination of MAI had been seen in fewer than 20 patients before the recognition of AIDS. AIDS patients tend to develop MAI infections more than ordinary tuberculosis. The immunologic defect in AIDS patients makes them more susceptible to this organism. In these patients, the disease is relentless in its devastation and involves not only the lung, but may also spread to the liver, spleen, lymph nodes, bone marrow, gastrointestinal tract, skin, and brain. Symptoms may include cough, shortness of breath, generalized debilitation with marked weight loss, severe diarrhea accompanied by abdominal pains, and lymph node enlargement (swollen glands). Involvement of the brain may give rise to a number of complaints such as headache, visual problems, weakness, and loss of balance.

Attempts to arrest the disease with antibiotic therapy have been unrewarding, only small gains having been made by the use of two new drugs—ansamycin, a derivative of the standard antituberculosis drug rifampin, and clofazimine, an antileprosy drug. Multiple-drug regimes employing combinations of 4 or 5 drugs simultaneously result in a limited containment of the disease. The recent discovery of a new penicillin-like drug (a "super" penicillin) named thienamycin, to be tested in conjunction with an already available antibiotic, amikacin, may hold promise in the treatment of MAI infections. The disease is also quite resistant to therapy in non-AIDS patients.

### Salmonella

Salmonella infections, like other opportunistic infections, are seen with increasing frequency in patients with a defect of cell-mediated immunity. Salmonellosis is one of the most common infections in the United States; over 2 million cases appear annually. It may present as a mild gastroenteritis, a localized infection, a brain infection, or a severe blood infection (e.g., typhoid fever). Symptoms are fever, abdominal pain, severe diarrhea, headaches, and rash. It is usually a benign disease that follows the ingestion of contaminated or inadequately prepared foods, especially eggs, chicken, and duck. In the homosexual population, it is acquired through anal-oral sexual activities.

Diagnosis depends on isolating the organism from blood or stools. Usually the intestinal infection is self-limiting and improves within a week, requiring only supportive treatment (e.g., fluids, rest, etc).

The treatment of typhoid fever, caused by *Salmonella typhii*, is difficult because the organism can reside in areas of the body not easily reached by antibiotics. It requires potent antibiotic therapy (ampicillin or chloramphenicol) for long periods of time.

## Nocardia

Nocardia are common soil organisms that grow in a branching fashion similar to fungi or mold. Nocardia infections are common in man, but usually cause severe pulmonary and disseminated disease only in those with compromised immune systems. In these patients, the disease usually begins as a lung infection that progresses to a collection of pus (abscess). Nocardial infections behave like other chronic lung infections, resulting in cough, sputum production, chest pain, fever, and generalized debilitation. If the infection travels in the blood to the brain, the patient may complain of confusion, dizziness, headaches, seizures, and other neurologic symptoms. Because of the nonspecific nature of the disease and its rarity, only a high degree of suspicion and appropriate laboratory tests establish the diagnosis. Treatment of nocardial disease may be extremely difficult, and prolonged use of antibiotics is often necessary. The prognosis is poor for any patient with this illness, but is especially grim if associated with AIDS.

## Listeria

*Listeria monocytogenes* is a bacterium that causes infection mostly in fetuses, neonates, the elderly, and immunocompromised patients. The very young and the very old are considered to be immunologically incompetent and therefore susceptible to opportunistic infections (e.g., by Listeria) traditionally seen in patients lacking immune defenses due to lymphoma, treatment to prevent rejection of a renal transplant, or other causes of T-cell deficiency. Listeria infection is transmitted to the fetus *in utero* (during the pregnancy) or at the time of passage through the birth canal. Older humans acquire this infection through inhaling contaminated dust or through contact with infected animals or contaminated sewage or soil. The majority of patients present with a severe brain infection characterized by fever, delirium, sometimes coma, convulsions and even shock. Diagnosis is made by a microscopic examination of body fluids. Cultures of blood and spinal fluids are sometimes revealing. Treatment consists of combinations of antibiotics such as penicillin, erythromycin, and ampicillin.

Dr. Donald B. Louria has suggested that this organism would be expected to cause disease in AIDS patients at a greater rate than in the general population, but, logical as this suggestion seems, Listeria infection is rare in AIDS patients. Only time and careful microbiological screening will establish or disprove the potential for infection with the Listeria organism.

**Other Bacterial Infections**

Two particular agents of bacterial pneumonia, *Hemophilus influenzae* and *Streptococcus pneumoniae*, are seen with greater frequency in AIDS patients than in the general population. Some AIDS patients with *Pneumocystis carinii* pneumonia have also had either pneumococcal or *H. influenzae* pneumonia. It is interesting to speculate that this conjunction of pneumonias may be due to an immunologic defect recently demonstrated by the National Institutes of Health in AIDS patients. Specifically, in addition to the T-cell defect discussed in detail in Chapter 3, there is a B-cell defect that influences antibody production. It is now known that AIDS patients have high levels of antibodies, proteins produced by B lymphocytes in response to the intrusion of "foreign material" (antigen). Antibody attacks the foreign material and helps to dispose of it or to reduce its harmful effect on the body. What appears to be unique to the AIDS patients is antibody that is ineffective or poorly functioning. The inability of the B cells to produce normally active antibody may possibly increase the AIDS patient's susceptibility to infection by common bacteria such as *Staphylococcus epidermidis*. These bacteria are one of the most common causes of hospital-acquired infection. *S. epidermidis* infections appear most often when foreign bodies are present, e.g., when intravenous catheters are inserted in blood vessels to infuse medicine, or when tubes are placed in the bladder to remove urinary waste. The most common presentation of *S. epidermidis* infection in this setting is that of blood infection, or sepsis, manifested as a high fever, sweating, fatigue, and general decline of the patient's health.

It will be interesting to learn the eventual importance of the bacteria discussed above in the overall clinical picture of AIDS infections. No doubt new associations of bacterial infection and AIDS will arise. Whatever the future may hold, one thing is frighteningly clear: Infections by bacteria such as MAI respond poorly to antibiotic treatment. Until we can reverse the immunodeficiency characteristic of AIDS, these infections will not be successfully treated with antibiotics alone.

## FUNGAL INFECTIONS

Fungi are microscopic organisms commonly found in nature in two principal forms, yeasts and molds. The simpler form is the yeasts, single-celled organisms that divide by budding small daughter cells. Yeasts are widespread in the environment and in baker's and brewer's yeasts.

Molds are composed of branching, intertwined cells that create the characteristic fuzzy appearance. A familiar mold is the one that grows on bread.

Most fungi, both yeasts and molds, do not cause human disease. When disease does occur, for example, fungal skin infections such as diaper rash and jock itch, it usually tends to be a nuisance rather than a threat. When fungi do cause serious infection, they do so primarily in individuals with an abnormal immune system, for example, in cancer patients or in patients receiving drugs that depress the immune system. Since AIDS patients characteristically have an impaired immune system, it is not at all surprising that they are candidates for certain fungal infections.

### Candida albicans

The most common fungal infection seen in AIDS patients is due to a yeast called *Candida albicans*. Indeed, some physicians consider it a clue to the presence of AIDS if found in the proper clinical setting. Fortunately, it is not typically a serious infection. Candida causes a superficial infection of the mouth and throat with pain and white plaques in the affected areas. Though it may be very difficult to cure in AIDS patients and tends to recur, it rarely spreads to other parts of the body and, therefore, is not likely to be fatal. Candida also causes infections in patients, e.g., diabetics, who do not have AIDS, and is responsible for certain types of diaper rash, oral thrush in infants, and vaginal infections in women.

Some groups that acquire similar superficial candida infections— AIDS patients and infants born with certain genetic immune deficiencies, glandular disturbances, or tumors—share in common an impaired T-cell immune system.

**Cryptococcus**

Another fungal infection seen in AIDS patients is due to Cryptococcus, another yeast common in nature, that causes disease in patients with immune defects. Cryptococcus produces a thick, protective capsule that enables it to resist the body's defenses. The yeast enters the body via the lungs, migrates into the blood, and spreads to other organs, especially the brain. In the brain, it causes severe meningitis, which is very resistant to therapy and often fatal.

**Histoplasma**

The third fungus seen in AIDS patients is called Histoplasma. This fungus is also very common in nature, especially in the Ohio River valley and eastern United States. People with normal immunity are commonly exposed to Histoplasma without developing disease. If disease does develop, it produces upper respiratory symptoms in healthy adults, but in AIDS patients it quickly involves the lung, liver, spleen, brain, and gastrointestinal tract. The increasing number of severe Histoplasma infections described in AIDS patients is again the consequence of their T-cell defect.

Diagnosis of Histoplasma infections is helped by recovery of the fungus from the blood, urine, or infected organ tissues. Amphotericin is used for treatment.

## SUMMARY

AIDS is characterized by a melange of rare bacterial and fungal diseases and disorders that are consequences of the body's frail and failing immune system. Immune dysfunction does not cause the deaths, but complications of the diseases do. The clinical course in these patients is marked by recurrent, severe, multiple opportunistic infections, which present major challenges to physician and patient alike. Treatment with antibiotics may temporarily control opportunistic infections, but merely postpones, rather than prevents, the development of other AIDS-related illnesses.

# 6     Cancers and AIDS
## MICHAEL NISSENBLATT

## KAPOSI'S SARCOMA

In 1872, Dr. Moriz Kaposi, a dermatologist, described a new disease. Three middle-aged men were found to have clusters of hard, round, nodular growths located, typically, around the hands and feet. These lesions were deeply pigmented and colored brownish-red or bluish-red due to bleeding within them. In addition to the deformity, the malady caused a feeling of tension and pain in the affected areas. It was also fatal; the first 2 patients died within 3 years of diagnosis as the malignancy slowly progressed to involve the lungs, liver, and other abdominal organs. The disease was subsequently termed Kaposi's sarcoma (KS).

KS was a rare disease. In the first 75 years after the initial description, only 500 cases were reported, and by 1960 a total of 1200 cases had been documented in the medical literature. The majority of patients were elderly men of eastern European, Italian, or Russian descent. Later, a more serious form of the disease was reported among black African children living in a region near the equator. The disease was uncommon in the United States, with only 2–6 cases reported per year for every 10 million Americans.

In the mid- and late 1970s, however, the incidence of the disease began to increase. It was reported among dialysis and kidney transplant patients, in individuals with cancer, and in patients receiving chemotherapy—drugs used in the treatment of cancer. And in 1979 it was reported for the first time in young homosexual males. The common characteristic among these groups was acquired immunodeficiency—an impairment of the immune system as a consequence of underlying illness.

## Signs and Symptoms

There are several forms of KS. The rarest, known as the lymph-node (lymphadenopathic) form, is an aggressive skin cancer that often spreads to other organs such as the lymph nodes, lung, bone, and bowel. This form was virtually unknown among practicing oncologists (cancer specialists) before AIDS appeared. Its signs and symptoms reflected the nature of the disease. For example, involvement of the glands (lymph nodes) can result in swelling of the armpits, groin, or neck. KS invasion of bone can cause fractures, pain, and even the release of calcium into the bloodstream. When the lungs are affected, the airways may be obstructed by tumor, or fluid may exude onto the surface of the lung (pleural effusion), resulting in shortness of breath and a cough productive of bloody sputum. About 40% of patients with this type of KS develop intestinal involvement, which can lead to blockage or hemorrhage of the bowel.

The most common variety of KS is limited to the skin. It is a slowly progressive malignancy occurring in elderly men. Since the average survival rate is 8–13 years, patients usually die from causes other than KS.

In recent years, however, the form of KS associated with AIDS has changed the usual course of this disease. This form is a more aggressive neoplasm, with a 40% mortality rate during the first year after diagnosis. AIDS-associated KS afflicts one-third of all AIDS patients.

## Etiology

Why do patients with AIDS develop KS? The cause of KS is unknown, but a multifactorial etiology is suspected, including environmental and genetic factors and infections. The clustering of KS in particular geographic areas suggests an environmental influence. Ethnic predispositions to KS, and the fact that patients with classic KS and AIDS patients with KS both have an increased incidence of a specific genetic marker called HLA-DR-5, suggest a hereditary or genetic influence.

AIDS patients develop numerous opportunistic infections, many of them viral. There are two major types of viruses. One is composed of RNA and the second of DNA. The majority of viruses causing infections in AIDS patients are composed of DNA and include herpes (types I and II), hepatitis B, non-A non-B hepatitis, and, most importantly, cytomegalovirus (CMV). One group of researchers confirmed that KS cells in the tissues of KS patients contained DNA from CMV. Other researchers have isolated CMV or antibodies to CMV in the blood of AIDS patients. The majority of homosexuals also have frequent CMV infections.

Recent reports suggest that reduced immunity plays a role in the development and course of KS. For example, an increased incidence of KS is seen in kidney transplant recipients and in patients on drugs that decrease their immunity. These findings establish a close relationship between the presence of KS and that of CMV and suggest that CMV may be the etiologic agent promoting KS development in individuals who are genetically predisposed and have frequent and persistent CMV infections.

**Treatment**

KS is a malignancy that arises in a setting of profound immunodeficiency. Treatment can, therefore, be two-pronged: agents can be used to enhance the immune system or to combat the cancer. Initial treatment, directed at the cancer, included radiotherapy, monochemotherapy (one drug), and polychemotherapy (more than one drug).

Radiation therapy is usually reserved for patients with only small amounts of disease. Radiation machines (linear accelerators or cobalt teletherapy units) are designed to treat small, localized areas of skin or bone. A newer type of radiation therapy applies electrons "topically," i.e., over the entire surface of the body of patients in whom KS has extensively infiltrated the skin. This form of radiation therapy does not penetrate the body deeply and therefore produces fewer side effects, but is ineffective against malignancies involving internal organs. Patients with extensive internal disease require chemotherapy—drugs used to combat cancer that are able to permeate the entire body.

Chemotherapeutic drugs are given either by mouth or injection and circulate throughout the bloodstream. In this way they reach all of the organs and, when effective, can kill cancer regardless of its location. They work by interfering with the growth and reproduction of the cancer cell. There are many classes of chemotherapy. Some, which function like antibiotics, inhibit the production of vital proteins necessary for the survival of cancer cells. Used against KS, they can cause the disease to regress in 35–90% of the patients.

Most effective are drugs that prevent cell division. One, vinblastine (Velban), is known as a "spindle inhibitor." It is an alkaloid, extracted from the periwinkle plant (*Vinca rosea*), that binds to tubulin, a cylinder-shaped protein inside cells. Tubulin forms a spindle-like structure and enables the division of one cell into two (mitosis). Binding of tubulin by vinblastine arrests cells at this crucial step and causes cell death. When used as a single agent in KS patients, vinblastine achieves an overall response rate of 37%, and in 5% the measurable disease entirely regresses (complete remission). Approximately 25% of AIDS patients treated with vinblastine for KS developed opportunistic infections because their already impaired immunity may be further compromised by such treatment.

Etoposide (VP-16) is another highly active agent against KS. It also is a plant alkaloid. It originates in the May apple (*Podophyllum peltatum*) and mandrake plants and was long used as a folk remedy for drug poisoning and constipation. Etoposide (VP-16) binds to tubulin at a different site than vinblastine and prevents cells from entering the division sequence, thus killing them at a pre-mitosis stage (prophase). When Etoposide is used as a single agent, 79% of patients respond and in 38% all measurable disease regresses. Opportunistic infections do occur, but in only 12% of AIDS patients.

Although single agents like vinblastine and Etoposide may produce dramatic responses in KS patients, such responses are often of brief duration. Therefore, combinations of agents have been given in an attempt to improve the quality of response and the length of survival.

One recent combination produced a response rate of 86% lasting an average of more than 14 months; a second caused remarkable improvement of symptoms in 78% of the treated patients. However, chemotherapy increased the already high susceptibility to opportunistic infections. In fact, patients aggressively treated with chemotherapy are more likely to die of opportunistic infections than of the cancer itself. While there is indeed effective chemotherapy, the drugs can be hazardous.

Medical scientists are also trying to use the body's natural immune defense system to control cancer. Newer and less toxic immunologic agents are being developed to correct the underlying immunodeficiency that makes its victims susceptible to KS and opportunistic infections, but only preliminary results are available. The agents include transfer factor, thymosin, and interferon (particularly a type known as recombinant leukocyte A). Of the first 12 patients evaluated after treatment with interferon, 5 had major responses and 3 experienced brief improvements. A recent and larger test of interferon achieved a response rate of 40% with complete remission in 23%. It was found that high doses of interferon were most effective and that opportunistic infections were uncommon, in contrast to the high risk of chemotherapy. Interferon caused the best responses in a limited group of tissues—skin, bowel, and lymph nodes. Response duration varied, but the average exceeded 13 months.

Other approaches to treating KS in AIDS patients are also being developed. Plasmapheresis, a technique for removing cells and proteins from blood, is used to remove suppressor cells ($T_8$ cytotoxic suppressor cells) in an effort to restore a more normal immunity. Similarly, pure antibodies, called monoclonal, have been developed against these suppressor cells and administered by injection to achieve the same result.

A substance known as interleukin-2 has been shown to reconstitute immune responses in several animal models. A phase-I (toxicity) trial has recently been completed, and clinical activity against KS is now being explored.

Other "biologic response modifiers" being studied include retinoids (13-Cis retinoic acid) and isoprinosine. Isoprinosine has been shown to correct immune defects in patients with the prodrome called AIDS-related complex (ARC), but improvement was incomplete for fully expressed AIDS and KS.

The newest approaches to the treatment of KS, e.g., bone marrow transplantation (BMT), are in their infancy. In BMT, a donor provides bone marrow to a recipient with an otherwise fatal illness such as aplastic anemia, leukemia, or immunodeficiency disease. The donor cells, presumably healthy, can grow in the recipient and restore the deficient elements. To date, only two AIDS patients have received BMT and data are preliminary. Whether the immunologic disorder and clinical course of AIDS will be altered by BMT remains to be determined.

## OTHER CANCERS OF AIDS

Patients with AIDS may have malignancies other than KS. The same etiologic mechanism(s) that predisposes them to KS could conceivably also allow other rare neoplasms to develop. Some homosexuals, not definitively diagnosed as AIDS victims, have a generalized enlargement of their lymph glands (lymphadenopathy) and are quite ill with symptoms such as fatigue (60%), skin rash (25%), muscle pain (35%), sweating (15%), as well as hair loss, weight loss, and diarrhea. They exhibit impairment of cell-mediated immunity, but somewhat less profound than that of overt AIDS. When these lymph nodes are removed and examined, they display a microscopic pattern known as hyperplasia—the lymphocytes in the glands are growing rapidly as if in an effort to ward off some invading pathogen. This wasting syndrome found in groups at high risk for developing AIDS has been given many names: prodromal AIDS, AIDS-related complex (ARC) and lymphadenopathy syndrome. Between 10% and 30% of these patients will go on to develop overt AIDS with accompanying opportunistic infections and malignancies.

### Lymphomas

AIDS patients also tend to develop lymphoma, a cancer of the lymphatic system. The lymphatic system is comprised of a network of glands (lymph nodes) and interconnecting vessels that manufacture and circulate lymph, a clear liquid containing lymphocytes (white blood cells). The lymphatic system plays an important role in fighting infection. Lymph nodes act as filters to trap dead cells, cell fragments, invading bacteria, and even cancer cells. They often become swollen and sore during an infection, e.g., the common "sore throat."

In AIDS, however, a rapid and uncontrolled growth of lymphocytes occurs within the lymph nodes, resulting in lymphomas. Lymphomas are divided into two major classes: Hodgkin's disease and non-Hodgkin's lymphomas. AIDS patients typically present with the latter.

Lymphomas are the second most common type of cancer found in AIDS, ultimately affecting 5–15% of AIDS patients. The earliest symptoms include painless enlargement of a lymph node or group of nodes, sometimes several separate clusters of nodes simultaneously, e.g., in the neck, armpits, and groin. Sometimes, the spleen and liver are also enlarged. As the lymphoma progresses, the patient develops symptoms specific to the area involved and may also complain of persistent fatigue, fever, night sweats, weight loss, nausea, vomiting, and abdominal pain. The lymphoma may spread to other parts of the lymphatic system and even to other tissues and organs. The malignancy results in a proliferation of abnormal lymphocytes that lack the usual ability to combat infections. As the disease progresses, the body is left with fewer red blood cells (anemia) and fewer normal, disease-fighting lymphocytes.

*Burkitt-like Lymphomas*
The majority of lymphomas in AIDS patients affect the B-lymphocyte population. They are called "Burkitt-like" lymphomas because of evidence suggesting some shared characteristic with the previously known Burkitt's lymphomas.

Burkitt's lymphomas are of two types: African Burkitt's, which usually invades the jaw, may distort the entire face, and can spread to other organs, and American Burkitt's, which spares the jaw and face but produces an abdominal tumor. In the United States, American Burkitt's has been considered uncommon, but is now being reported in increasing numbers in AIDS patients.

The cause of Burkitt's lymphoma is probably the herpes-like Epstein-Barr virus, identified by electron microscopy in most African Burkitt's patients and in some American cases. Tissue samples from American and African Burkitt's patients appear identical under the microscope.

Some interrelationship between these lymphomas and AIDS is likely. In an equatorial region, where black African children have a high incidence of KS, there is also a high incidence of African Burkitt's lymphoma. Also, like AIDS patients, African children with KS have generally been infected with CMV, too, and those with African Burkitt's lymphoma have been infected with the Epstein-Barr virus.

In a collective study, the average age of 90 AIDS patients with Burkitt-like lymphoma was 37 years. Seventy-five of the patients were known to have had ARC or overt AIDS before the lymphoma was diagnosed; in the remaining 15, the immunodeficiency was silent and the malignancy was the presenting feature. These lymphomas were biologically aggressive.

*Lymphoblastic Lymphomas*
A second type of lymphoma, usually rare but already reported in at least 10 AIDS cases, attacks the brain and frequently invades the bone marrow. It is called lymphoblastic lymphoma. Patients may complain of headaches, visual disturbances, nausea, vomiting, confusion, weakness, and other neurologic symptoms. CAT scans can reveal a mass in the brain, and microscopic examination of brain tissue confirms the lymphoma.

Why are lymphomas so common in AIDS? Dr. Robert Gallo and a team of researchers recently isolated a retrovirus, called human T-cell leukemia/lymphoma virus (HTLV-III), in lymph nodes from patients with the gay-lymph-node syndrome (lymphadenopathy) and ARC. Antibodies to HTLV-III have also been found in the majority of AIDS and ARC patients. Thus, HTLV-III is a likely candidate for the cause of AIDS. Indeed, HTLV-III is attracted to helper T lymphocytes (T-cells) and causes them to express on their surfaces a receptor for a growth-promoting substance called T-cell growth factor (TCGF), which confers a degree of immortality upon the infected cells. Hence, observation in the laboratory of enhanced lymphocyte growth and activation (lymphoblastogenesis) may reflect the clinical expression of lymphadenopathy or malignant lymphoma.

**Treatment of Lymphomas**

Once a lymphoma diagnosis is established, an elaborate sequence of investigations is performed to determine the extent of spread to other organs. This process is called staging. If only one or two sites are found to be involved, the disease is said to be at stage I or II, which often responds to aggressive radiation treatment delivered to all the affected sites at once. However, when the disease is detected in multiple locations, or in visceral organs (e.g., liver, lung, or bone marrow), it is at advanced stage III or IV and requires general chemotherapy rather than localized radiation.

Drugs are given in combination—as many as 3 to 8 different agents—to take advantage of their highly specialized modes of action. Combinations known as CHOP (Cytoxan, hydroxydavnoru-bicin, Oncovin, and prednisone) and CHOP-BLEO (CHOP-bleo-mycin) are particularly popular because they produce a complete remission (disease-free state) in 50–75% of patients and a cure (permanent disease-free state) in up to 30%. A newer regimen—PROMALE-MOPP (prednisone, methotrexate, Adriamycin, Cytoxan, Etoposide—mustard, Oncovin, procarbazine, prednisone)—offers still greater promise.

### Hodgkin's Disease

Hodgkin's disease was not associated with AIDS until 7 such cases were recently identified at Stanford. All had advanced disease. Quite remarkably, skin and extensive intra-abdominal involvement were found, unusual features in Hodgkin's disease but typical of the Burkitt-like lymphoma of AIDS.

### Cancers of Sexually Traumatized Tissues

AIDS patients may also develop cancers of tissues traumatized during sexual activity, including the anus, rectum, and throat. Because of proximity to the anus, cancer of the rectum usually presents with rectal pain and bleeding. If the tumor is advanced, it may obstruct the bowel. Interestingly, it is known that viral infections may cause these cancers. Types I and II herpes have long been associated with cancers of the throat and rectum, respectively. Experience in managing these tumors, however, is limited. For cancer of the rectum, and often of the anus, the rectum is usually removed and the bowel re-attached to the outer wall of the abdomen (colostomy) to discharge waste into a drainage bag. However, recent advances in radiation treatments and chemotherapy have been increasingly curative, even without surgery.

### NONMALIGNANT NEOPLASMS

Finally, there is growing evidence of an increased frequency of non-malignant neoplasms in AIDS patients. For example, angiolipomas, common benign tumors originating in fat (adipose) tissue usually account for 5–17% of all fatty tumors. Recently, however, of 8 angio-lipomas removed within a short period at one institution, 7 came from homosexual men, and no other type of fatty tumor was noted in the homosexual group over a 5-month interval. To date, no unusual behavior has been attributed to these lesions. The main concern is the occasional confusion of angiolipomas with KS.

## SUMMARY

AIDS patients are susceptible to a variety of malignancies, the most common of which is Kaposi's sarcoma (KS). Until the appearance of AIDS, KS had been rare, primarily affecting elderly men of Mediterranean descent and usually causing little or no pain or complications. However, the KS that affects AIDS patients is very aggressive, involving the skin, lymph nodes, and abdominal organs. Other malignancies also are found in AIDS victims and include lymphomas and cancers of the anus, rectum, and throat. Treatment of these cancers is possible and may in immunocompetent individuals achieve remission or cure. However, their aggressive nature in conjunction with the variety of opportunistic infections that AIDS patients also develop makes treatment especially complex. AIDS patients may respond to various cancer modalities, including radiotherapy, chemotherapy, and immunotherapy, but the underlying immunodeficiency typically results in the development of multiple and recurrent infections and other malignancies.

# Three  Implications

# 7    The Elusive Etiology—
## Possible Causes and
## Pathogenesis of AIDS
### EDWARD JOHNSON AND PETER HO

The understanding and conquest of more recently recognized diseases such as Legionnaires disease, toxic shock syndrome, and hepatitis B are made possible by lessons learned in the campaigns against such older infectious diseases as cholera, smallpox, plague, and tuberculosis. Such lessons were based on slowly and painfully acquired bodies of basic and clinical knowledge. Often, the spread of the diseases was arrested long before the causative organisms were isolated. A good example is cholera. After a severe outbreak of cholera in London, England in 1832, John Snow was able to halt its advance by means of a careful epidemiologic study before the establishment of the germ theory and several decades before the etiology of cholera was found.

A decade ago, Legionnaires disease, toxic shock syndrome, and AIDS were unknown. A question immediately comes to mind: Are we giving old diseases new names or suddenly confronting an array of microbes never encountered before? Legionella is now known to have caused several outbreaks of pneumonia and other ailments that preceded isolation of the organism by several decades. Frozen serum samples stored long ago by some farsighted epidemiologists made possible the discovery of this important information with the aid of modern techniques using serum antibody specific for the legionella bacteria. Toxic shock syndrome was variously described long before it became a distinct clinical entity. Now the acquired immune deficiency syndrome (AIDS) has caused great excitement among the public and the scientific community, in part due to its multifaceted and problematic elements.

Solutions to the AIDS enigma are being sought by medical detectives, like those at the Centers for Disease Control. These researchers hope to unravel the puzzle by isolating the putative "AIDS agent." When found, the agent must be shown to fulfill Koch's postulates: it must be isolated in all affected individuals, it must be grown in pure culture, and the disease must be reproduced in experimental animals.

Treatment and cure of AIDS depend upon elucidation of its etiology. Three major hypotheses have been proposed: immune overload, single infectious agent, and multifactorial. The immune overload hypothesis suggests that AIDS is caused by repeated exposure to infections, toxins, antigens, and lifestyle factors that create a predisposition to the disease. The multiple and persistent challenges to the immune system result in a paralysis of the body's defense against pathogens. The single infectious agent hypothesis proposes that a single agent causes severe immunosuppression, creating a vulnerability to opportunistic infections and malignancies. The multifactorial hypothesis holds that AIDS may be the result of a sequence of immune-system defects and reactivation of a latent viral infection.

**IMMUNE-OVERLOAD HYPOTHESIS**

The immune-overload hypothesis was the earliest to be advanced, largely due to the recognition of AIDS in the homosexual population. This group is of particular interest to the medical community because it exhibits a high incidence of sexually transmitted diseases (STDs). During the 1970s, physicians became aware of new STDs in the gay community and the community's unique medical needs. Special clinics were developed to treat and chronicle infections that plagued this segment of the population. Terms such as "gay bowel" and "gay bar" syndrome emerged to describe particular patterns of disease, specifically rectal discharge, with or without pain, and the isolation of bacteria, parasites, and viruses that, until recently, rarely caused lower bowel infections.

Physicians, previously unaware of the degree of promiscuity in some parts of the gay world, were astounded and challenged by patients often presenting with 3 to 5 different, or new, STDs at one time. At least one homosexual male was documented as having 9 different, concomitant STDs. The widespread use of such drugs as amyl nitrite, butyl nitrite, amphetamines, Quaaludes, cocaine, and heroin, in conjunction with the sexual use of foreign bodies and fists, rectal intercourse, and, in particular, "rimming" (oral-anal sex), has led many investigators to favor the immune overload hypothesis.

Part of this hypothesis attributes central significance to the many viruses common to homosexuals, drug addicts, hemophiliacs, and immune-compromised individuals such as organ transplant recipients and those undergoing chemotherapy for cancer. These viruses are all suspect as potential etiologic agents for AIDS. Of the immunosuppressive factors and agents that have been documented or proposed, the following are of great importance.

**Repeated Infections**

AIDS patients have shown evidence of an impaired immune system even before developing the syndrome. It is suggested that the opportunistic infections that abound in these patients are the result of a chronically overloaded or exhausted immune system. The high-risk groups, especially promiscuous homosexuals and intravenous-drug abusers, are characteristically infected, either sequentially or simultaneously, with multiple infectious agents.

**Intravenous Narcotic Drugs**

Narcotic drugs have been known to cause immune defects in both humans and experimental animals. There is marked suppression of T lymphocytes, leading to defective cellular immunity, and stimulation of the B lymphocytes results in an increased production of antibodies (immunoglobulins). It has been speculated that defective cellular immunity and disturbances of humoral immunity may contribute to the increased frequency of viral and bacterial infections seen in intravenous-drug abusers. Furthermore, chronic intravenous-drug abuse may involve multiple organ systems, including the heart, lungs, liver, and lymphatic system, causing diffuse enlargement of lymph nodes.

This may contribute to further deterioration of the body's defense system against infections.

### Nitrite Inhalation

The use of amyl nitrite, or "poppers," as a sexual stimulant has been widely practiced among many homosexuals since the 1960s. Amyl nitrite and the related compound isobutyl nitrite can cause immunosuppression, as evidenced by an increase in suppressor T cells and a decrease in helper T cells. A study reported in Lancet (1982) noted that the lowest ratios of helper to suppressor T cells were found in homosexuals who were regular nitrite users. However, conflicting reports in subsequent clinical investigations clouded the role of nitrites in the development of AIDS, and nitrite usage is closely linked to other variables that are also possible causative agents of AIDS, e.g., certain homosexual practices, meeting places, other drugs, and sexually transmitted infections. The occurrence of AIDS among populations that do not use nitrite inhalants argues against this drug as the etiologic agent, but does not exclude it from some role in the development of AIDS illnesses.

### Sperm

A promiscuous homosexual lifestyle has consistently been shown to be the major risk factor in the development of AIDS. The extensive sexual activity of a subset of male homosexuals is truly amazing—some have over 1,000 different sexual partners in a lifetime. It is well known that sperm has profound effects on the immune system. For example, recent studies have shown that, even in healthy homosexuals, sperm impairs the immune system, although less severely than in those with AIDS. Injection of sperm into laboratory animals causes a marked humoral immune response and cellular immune suppression. Those who practice passive (receptive) anal intercourse have significantly higher numbers of suppressor T cells than do those who practice only active (insertive) anal intercourse.

A recent prominent theory on the etiology of AIDS implicates a virus in the semen of homosexual males that primarily affects the T and B lymphocytes. Anal intercourse frequently tears the mucosa of the rectum and may permit direct entry of sperm into blood vessels. Sperm is normally shielded from the immune system and does not enter the blood stream. When it does gain entry into the circulation, it is perceived by the body as a foreign substance (nonself), an antigen, and the body produces antibodies against it. Repeated exposure of the immune system to sperm and the production of antisperm antibodies is believed by some, but not all, researchers to be an important risk factor in the ultimate expression of AIDS among homosexuals. However, homosexuality is not new to mankind, and cannot therefore be acclaimed as the sole etiologic source of AIDS.

**Genetic Predisposition**

Genetic predisposition is known to be important in many diseases such as lupus and diabetes. Although it probably is not the cause, it is thought by some investigators to be a factor in the development of AIDS. A specific genetic marker termed HLA-DR5 (HLA stands for human leukocyte antigen) is frequently found among homosexual men with Kaposi's sarcoma (KS). Interestingly, homosexual men with KS are frequently of Italian origin, and Italians have a relatively high frequency of HLA-DR5.

HLAs, discovered in the 1950s, were isolated from white blood cells where they reside. When an individual is exposed to foreign cells, the most important immune response is against HLAs. The HLA system has proved to be very useful in tissue typing for organ transplantation. For example, for a kidney transplant, the closer the HLA matching between the donor and recipient, the higher the chance of a successful transplant. Many diseases have been found to be related to the HLA system, including KS. Since many individuals may have been exposed to the AIDS agent, but only a small percentage develop AIDS, genetic factors may predispose some groups to the disease. However, it is doubtful that genetic factors alone can cause AIDS.

## SINGLE-AGENT HYPOTHESIS

The possible etiological agents of AIDS that have received the most attention are viruses. These have been widely documented as the cause of disease and immunosuppression in homosexuals, drug addicts, hemophiliacs, Haitians, patients who have received transplanted organs, and patients with T-cell defects known to be caused by certain tumors. That these viruses can cause disease in individuals not at risk for AIDS is undeniable; it is the frequency and severity of the disease in high-risk populations that is of special concern. The possible existence of previously undetected agents, new activity of viruses that formerly caused disease only in animals, "mutated," more virulent strains, or subunits of already known agents have all been considered and deserve mention. New viruses are continually being isolated as culture techniques improve; viruses once thought to cause disease only in animals, both domesticated and wild, are more frequently being shown to cause disease in humans; and relatively benign viruses with altered genetic material are suspected of giving rise to severe infection in man and animals. Technological advances now allow scientists to identify the structure of these viral pathogens. The following is a summary of the arguments for and against a new disease agent.

| Arguments for a New Agent | Arguments Against a New Agent |
| --- | --- |
| Syndrome not known to exist prior to 1978 | No single agent isolated from all AIDS patients (including HTLV) |
| Differences of lifestyle in high-risk groups (homosexuals, drug addicts, Haitians, hemophiliacs) | Failure to produce AIDS in animals injected with blood and other tissues from AIDS patients |
| Cluster outbreaks of the disease (especially N.Y.C., L.A., S.F.) | Nearly all gay men with AIDS have antibodies against CMV (but a high rate exists among healthy gay men as well) |
| Epidemiologic studies showing chains of sexual contact in AIDS patients greater than expected by chance | No single strain of CMV detected in AIDS victims |
| AIDS risk groups especially subject to hepatitis B, suggesting similar type of transmission | Endemic population with HTLV free of AIDS (Japan) |
| Isolation of HTLV, a possible new agent, at roughly the same time AIDS epidemic began | |
| HTLV common in geographical areas where KS is epidemic and also in the Caribbean (Haitian connection) | |

In addition to viruses, we must consider nonviral agents as possible contributors to or causes of AIDS. Several viral and nonviral candidates are considered below, together with factors that make them possible causes and not just secondary or opportunistic infections in AIDS victims.

### Cytomegalovirus

Cytomegalovirus (CMV) disease was first documented in association with a high incidence of infection among gay men in San Francisco in 1979. This virus has been known to cause a spectrum of illnesses ranging from clinically silent infections to overwhelming and life-threatening disease, especially in immunocompromised patients. Transmission of CMV is also associated with intravenous-drug abuse.

Patients who receive transplanted organs require immunosuppressive therapy, drugs that blunt the immune system to prevent it from attacking the transplanted organ as foreign material. Almost always, these patients become infected with CMV and then other opportunistic infections and tumors. This has been proposed by many to be the sequence of events in AIDS patients. Unfortunately for AIDS patients, their immunosuppression cannot be turned off as it can be in renal transplant patients merely by discontinuing or decreasing the administration of immunosuppressive drugs. Other evidence linking CMV and AIDS is the epidemiologic and genetic connections between CMV and KS in AIDS patients. CMV has been shown to actually insert its DNA genetic material into KS tissue. CMV has repeatedly been isolated from KS patients' blood, urine, and body tissue.

It has been argued, however, that the presence of CMV in AIDS patients is only the result of immunosuppression and reactivation of a previous CMV infection. That is, many viruses, and in particular the herpesviruses of which CMV is a member, can rest dormant in patients' cells. Certain factors, such as immunosuppression, can periodically "awaken" these viruses. Once the virus is allowed or forced to become active, it begins to multiply and cause disease. Another argument against CMV as the cause of AIDS is the possibility that this virus is only a contaminant of the KS tissues from which it has been isolated. It can be reasoned that a virus like CMV, which is so prevalent in nature and especially so in populations at risk for AIDS, could easily contaminate tissue specimens. Since CMV has been known for some time to cause disease with certain characteristics, why should it suddenly start now to behave differently? This question recurs for other agents to be discussed.

### Epstein-Barr Virus

Like CMV, the Epstein-Barr virus (EBV) produces illnesses that range from subclinical to overwhelming infections, especially among immunoincompetent patients. EBV has also been implicated in malignancies such as African Burkitt's lymphoma and nasopharyngeal carcinoma. The prodromal phase of AIDS is typified by a viral-like illness reminiscent of infectious mononucleosis (caused by EBV) and may consist of malaise, fever, sweats, swollen glands (which may be chronic), enlarged spleen and liver, and changes in the immune system similar to those seen in AIDS.

EBV is common in all populations known to be at risk for AIDS (as evidenced by laboratory tests indicating past infection), and studies of gay men reveal that essentially 100% have had past infection. In AIDS patients the rate of reactivation of EBV infection is high (about 33%), and many victims have a history of recent episodes of EBV-mononucleosis prior to the diagnosis of AIDS. Again, as with CMV, the question is why should a well-delineated disease begin to behave in a different and more aggressive manner in the absence of evidence that any new strains or mutations have developed?

### Hepatitis B

Experience with hepatitis B has provided a model for the infectious pattern of a potential AIDS agent. The unfolding of the AIDS story is likely to follow the hepatitis B pattern in which the clinical presentation, incubation period, and probable routes of transmission were well understood for more than 10 years before the virus was finally identified. The extraordinarily high rate of current or past hepatitis B infections in the gay male and intravenous-drug abuser, combined with obviously possible routes of transmission of the disease (needlestick, blood products, sexual contacts), made the hepatitis B virus a particularly good candidate for an AIDS agent. This was bolstered by the fact that a specific subunit of hepatitis B (the delta particle) was isolated about the same time that AIDS first appeared. The delta particle has proved not to be a cause of AIDS, but the possible existence of another, still undetected subunit cannot be ruled out.

Hepatitis B subunits represent only a part of the virus from which they are derived. They can be transmitted from host to host as particles independent of the parent virus and exert their separate influence because they contain bits of DNA. Undoubtedly, new viral subunits will be isolated in the near future, and it is essential to remember that their DNA content may potentially be rearranged. That is, the information encoded in the DNA may be different from that of the parent virus. Thus, a pathogenic fragment of the parent virus may produce a different disease.

The predominant obstacle to the feasibility of hepatitis B as a cause of AIDS lies in the fact that hospital personnel, especially those who work directly with AIDS patients, have not contracted AIDS. Although health-care personnel are known to have suffered finger sticks with needles contaminated with body secretions from AIDS patients, none have gone on to develop AIDS, even after a 2-year incubation period. The absence of AIDS among these individuals lends support to the concept that multiple factors are involved in the pathogenesis of AIDS, and that repeated exposure or contact with extremely large quantities of infected material may be necessary to produce the syndrome.

**Parvovirus**

Parvoviruses are tiny DNA viruses that cause infections in many different species of animals. Past studies of parvoviruses were largely concerned with the economic import of infected animals, how the viruses infect their hosts, and the viruses' effect on the immune system. These viruses, through the expression of the diseases they cause in mink, dogs, mice, and other species, demonstrate several characteristics that could be important in the causation of AIDS. Specifically, they "jump" from one species to another (most viruses are species-specific and do not transfer from one kind of animal to another); they are able to alter their genetic material and progress from a noninfective to an infective state; and they have a propensity for causing not only a change in the infected animal's immune status but, in particular, a change in T-cell function. In addition, parvoviruses, like CMV and EBV, have been associated with tumors.

**Retroviruses: Human T-Cell Leukemia Viruses**

Much excitement has been generated by the discovery of various retroviruses in some AIDS patients. These retroviruses had previously been associated with tumors common to certain animals (feline leukemia) and to humans in particular geographic locations (Kyushu Island, Japan and the Caribbean, including Haiti). Central to the rapid sequence of events concerning these retroviruses are Dr. Robert Gallo of the National Cancer Institute in the United States and Dr. Luc Montagnier of the Pasteur Institute in France. These two men and their institutes form the "French connection" of AIDS.

Retroviruses are tiny, RNA-containing viruses first discovered in 1909 and shown by 1911 to have tumor-causing potential. In 1976, Dr. Gallo discovered a T-cell growth factor (TCGF) now called Interleukin-2 (IL-2). IL-2 is necessary for growing T cells in the laboratory and thus for isolating the retroviruses that may infect those cells. On the basis of the breakthrough with IL-2, Dr. Gallo was able to isolate the first human T-cell leukemia virus (HTLV-I) in 1982. HTLV-II was later isolated from a patient with a rare blood disease (hairy-cell leukemia). The occasional isolation of these HTLVs from patients with AIDS was of interest but, since they were not present as often as CMV, EBV, and hepatitis B, they were not likely to be the cause of AIDS. However, it was clear to many researchers that another, as yet unidentified retrovirus might be the causative agent of AIDS or at least a contributing factor. Retroviruses did, in fact, selectively attack T cells. They did cause immunological diseases in animals and man. They could be transmitted by sexual contact or blood products. Further, serological studies had shown that, even though most AIDS patients did not harbor HTLV-I or II, there was often evidence of exposure to an HTLV.

Technical advances have now made it possible to maintain a laboratory cell-line based on a cell isolated from an infected patient so that the continued growth of AIDS-related viruses can be studied. In late 1983, Dr. Gallo thus isolated HTLV-III from patients with AIDS and Dr. Montagnier isolated the lymphadenopathy associated virus (LAV) from a patient with the pre-AIDS lymphadenopathy syndrome. Present evidence strongly suggests that HTLV-III and LAV may actually be the same retrovirus and may cause or contribute to AIDS as part of, or as the result of, an immune overload.

## MULTIFACTORIAL HYPOTHESIS

One of the chief proponents of the multifactorial hypothesis is Dr. Joseph A. Sonnabend, who postulated a sequence of contributory steps to AIDS in a recent paper published in the Journal of the American Medical Association. The sequence begins with a reversible phase characterized by defective regulation of T cells caused by exposure to infectious agents, especially CMV and sperm. Defective T-cell regulation then permits reactivation of a latent EBV infection. The EBV stimulates B cells to increase the production of antibodies. The presence of large amounts of different antibodies may then induce autoimmune diseases such as a low white blood cell count, a low platelet count, rashes, and others. Sperm antibodies, in particular, may interact with antigens found on T-helper and other lymphocytes such as natural killer cells. This results in regulatory disturbances of the immune system and an inability to clear cells infected with herpesvirus. Furthermore, repeated exposure to other infections, the use of recreational drugs, and the influence of hereditary and environmental factors eventually lead to the final consequence of severe immune-function suppression.

The major shortcoming of the multifactorial hypothesis is that not all AIDS patients satisfy its requirements. Some homosexual men have developed AIDS with only limited sexual exposure, and AIDS has occurred in hemophiliacs, heterosexuals, recipients of blood transfusions, Haitians, and even children. Consequently, most investigators postulate an infectious agent, transmitted much like hepatitis B, as the probable cause of AIDS.

### PRESENT STATUS

Although HTLV-III and LAV are promising candidates for the cause of AIDS, many in the scientific community remain skeptical, and intense research continues. Nevertheless, the known facts indicate a syndrome that is well characterized clinically, epidemiologically, and immunologically. On the basis of present knowledge, it should be possible to confine the spread of the disease without being certain of its precise cause.

Whether or not the immune-overload, single-virus, or multifactorial hypothesis is accepted, it is universally agreed that promiscuity is a major risk factor, at least in the United States, and 90% of AIDS patients are homosexual or bisexual men and/or intravenous-drug abusers. Of course, if the single-virus view proves to be correct, and the pathogen is identified beyond doubt, then the fears of the public at large can be allayed and an immunologic approach would be the next logical step toward AIDS prevention. However, confirmation of such a finding may be laborious.

Meanwhile, properly designed clinical and epidemiologic studies must continue to resolve the question of whether AIDS poses a significant threat to the general public not now at high risk. More work is needed to clarify the risk of AIDS in blood transfusions and in immune defects induced by transfusions; the prognosis for otherwise healthy homosexuals, intravenous-drug abusers, and hemophiliacs who have T-lymphocyte abnormalities and generalized lymphadenopathy (swollen glands); and the possible influence of a genetic predisposition.

A marker to permit rapid diagnosis would be highly desirable. Of those being studied, none appear promising because they may be general indicators of previous infections rather than specific for AIDS. In this regard, the finding of antibodies to HTLV-III in both pre-AIDS and AIDS patients, if confirmed, is encouraging. Also, the experimental transmission of AIDS from 2 rhesus monkeys dying of the disease to 4 healthy monkeys may provide an animal model of great value for an understanding of the etiology of AIDS, since there have been few reports of AIDS in monkeys.

While awaiting further progress, the public not now at high risk can find comfort in the fact that no case of AIDS has been documented in health-care workers who did not have a previously weakened immune system. A concentrated effort to accurately and objectively educate the public about the epidemiological facts would go a long way to stem hysteria and to slow the spread of AIDS among high-risk groups by demonstrating the value of changing harmful personal habits. There are already gratifying signs that these groups are modifying their lifestyle.

## SUMMARY

The search for causes of outbreaks of "new infections" has always been exciting, frustrating, at times misdirected, and at times illuminating. AIDS has been no exception. The study of this disease during the last 4 years has been rewarded with a great advance toward an understanding of the immune system in health and disease. We have also gained invaluable knowledge concerning the natural history of many of the opportunistic infections associated with AIDS and T-cell deficiency in general. Presently, there is little doubt that HTLV-III is intimately related to the causation of AIDS. What is not clear is the exact nature of events leading to infection. Specifically, what infection(s) or condition(s) are necessary for the HTLV-III virus to attack the T-Helper cell and cause the immunologic devastation that is AIDS? It is here that the overwhelming question remains: Is the general population at risk in the future?

# 8        The Haitian Link

## JEFFREY VIEIRA

During the summer of 1982, investigators in Brooklyn, New York, and Miami, Florida, reported observations of 40 recent Haitian immigrants with unusual or opportunistic infections and/or Kaposi's sarcoma (KS). These cases had striking similarities to those described earlier among homosexuals and intravenous-narcotics abusers with the acquired immune deficiency syndrome (AIDS). Since Haitians lacked any of the then recognized risk factors for AIDS (e.g., promiscuous homosexual activity or intravenous-drug abuse), they were classified by the Centers for Disease Control (CDC) as a discrete high-risk group. The disease has subsequently been identified among severe hemophiliacs, spouses of AIDS victims, and newborns of mothers with clinical AIDS or risk factors for the disease. To date, the link between Haitians and others at risk remains unclear.

## EPIDEMIOLOGY

Between June 1981 and September 1983, 124 Haitian-Americans and 61 Haitians in Haiti (Pape et al., 1983) were identified who conform to the CDC case definition of AIDS. Reviews of hospital records and autopsy materials in Haiti have indicated that the onset of the epidemic there coincided with the first cases observed among homosexuals in New York and Los Angeles.

Haitian AIDS cases represent about 5% of the total in the United States, and this proportion has remained constant since 1982. They are for the most part recent immigrants, having lived in the United States an average of 2½ years prior to the onset of AIDS. Women constitute 7% of the cases among Haitian-Americans, which contrasts sharply with the situation in Haiti where as many as 25% of AIDS patients are women. The majority of patients are of lower socioeconomic status, although representatives of all strata have been afflicted.

## CLINICAL MANIFESTATIONS

The clinical presentation of AIDS in Haitians is similar to that of others at risk for acquiring the disease. The enlarged lymph nodes (lymphadenopathy), fever, weight loss, and chronic diarrhea which have become known as the AIDS prodrome or AIDS-related complex, are almost universal precursors of the disease. These signs and symptoms may persist for weeks to months before being recognized as opportunistic infections or malignancies.

Parasitic infections of the lung due to the protozoan *Pneumocystis carinii* and infection of the mouth and esophagus (oroesophagitis) due to the fungus *Candida albicans* are the most common opportunistic infections encountered in Haitians with AIDS, whether in the United States or Haiti. Certain infections appear to be particularly common in Haitian patients (when compared to non-Haitian patients), reflecting the endemicity of these pathogens in Haiti.

Disseminated *Mycobacterium tuberculosis* (TB) is the most common infection, and is found in about 50% of Haitians with AIDS (unpublished figures, New York City Department of Health). Because TB occurs sporadically in hosts with normal immunity, it is not considered an opportunistic infection by the CDC case definition. AIDS patients with TB can be differentiated from otherwise healthy TB patients by the presence in AIDS of significant depression of the cell-mediated immune system (Frank et al., 1983). This defect is best reflected by a reversal of the ratio of T-helper to T-suppressor cells and by the inability of the patient to respond with local swelling when challenged with skin-test antigens (PPD, Tine, mumps, Candida, and Trichophyton) injected under the superficial layers of the skin. Homosexuals and addicts with AIDS also develop mycobacterial infections, but these are usually caused by one of the so-called atypical mycobacteria, particularly *Mycobacterium avium-intracellulare*.

As many as 20% of Haitians with AIDS develop central nervous system (CNS) disease due to the parasite *Toxoplasma gondii* (unpublished figures, New York City Department of Health). The clinical presentation may take the form of meningitis, confusion and behavioral changes, or other neurological symptoms that mimic a stroke. The infection usually represents reactivation of latent (dormant) toxoplasmosis stimulated by the loss of effective cellular immune surveillance. In contrast to its incidence in Haitians with AIDS, *T. gondii* infections have been reported in fewer than 5% of non-Haitian victims.

Intestinal infections with parasites, such as amebiasis, giardiasis, and cryptospiridiosis, may be the cause of significant morbidity as a result of dehydrating fluid losses and malabsorption of nutrients; virtually 100% of AIDS patients in Haiti develop chronic diarrhea, often due to one or more of these parasites (Pape et al., 1983). Parasitic infections become less common in Haitian-Americans the longer they reside in the United States.

The characteristic laboratory profile of AIDS—anemia, decreased numbers of white blood cells (especially lymphocytes), decreased numbers of functional T-helper cells, and reversal of the T-helper/suppressor-cell ratio—is demonstrable in all Haitians with AIDS. As with homosexuals and many narcotics addicts, serologic studies reveal that most of the Haitians show evidence of previous infections with syphilis and viruses (Epstein-Barr, cytomegalovirus, herpes simplex, hepatitis A, and hepatitis B).

The overall mortality for AIDS at one year is 40–45%. In contrast, the one-year mortality for Haitian-Americans approaches 60%, and is over 70% in Haiti. This unfavorable prognosis is attributable to several factors. Malnutrition in rural Haiti is common (Lundahl, 1979). Recurrent or chronic parasitic infection combines with protein-calorie malnutrition to debilitate the patient and impair immune responses to serious infection. A minority of Haitian-Americans were malnourished prior to the onset of AIDS, but inanition (exhaustion induced by undernourishment) is the rule as the disease progresses. Also, although basic medical care is free in Haiti, the cost of medications is usually borne by the patient or his family. Because most patients with AIDS require prolonged therapy with antibiotics that are frequently expensive, some can afford only abbreviated courses of medication while others receive no therapy at all. The high incidence of CNS toxoplasmosis, with a mortality rate in excess of 75%, also elevates the overall mortality figures for this group.

## ETIOLOGY

It is hypothesized that AIDS is due to an infectious agent, most likely a virus, transmitted in a manner similar to hepatitis B, i.e., via blood, secretions, or sexual contact. The incubation period for this presumptive AIDS agent may be as long as months or years. Homosexuals are exposed to the agent by promiscuous sexual activity, intravenous-drug users by sharing of contaminated needles, hemophiliacs and other suspected transfusion-related cases by infusion of contaminated blood or blood components (such as antihemophilic Factors X and VIII), and spouses of victims by heterosexual contact and infected secretions.

From the outset, the mystery surrounding AIDS among Haitians has consisted of the lack of identifiable characteristics of Haitian lifestyle that would make Haitians more vulnerable to transmission of an infectious agent. Several clues have recently been uncovered through studies in the United States and, more importantly, in Haiti itself. A key observation has been that Haitians in general, and Haitians with AIDS in particular, have a high prevalence of markers (antibody and antigen) in their blood for hepatitis B virus (Pitchenik et al., 1983; Pape et al., 1983). This denotes widespread exposure to infected blood and/or secretions. Before exploring further the various theories of transmission among Haitians, it is worthwhile considering the social, economic, and cultural climate of Haiti.

Haiti occupies the western half of the island of Hispaniola in the Caribbean. It is the most densely populated and poorest nation in the Western Hemisphere. Its population is about 6 million. The natives are descended from central and western African blacks of various tribal origins brought to Haiti (then Saint Domingue) as slaves in the sixteenth and seventeenth centuries. French is the official language but Creole, a dialect unique to Haiti, is spoken by all natives.

Haiti is predominantly agrarian. Apart from a small middle and upper class of professionals and skilled technicians, the majority of the population achieves only a meager existence as common laborers or farmers. The mean annual income is less than $350. Since the mid-1960s, thousands of Haitians have emigrated to the United States and Canada to escape political repression. More recent emigrants, however, have been motivated by unfavorable economic conditions in Haiti. The majority of Haitians have settled in Miami, New York, and Newark, with smaller enclaves in Boston, Los Angeles, and Montreal. The population of Haitians in the United States is estimated at about 500,000, but this figure is imprecise due to the large number of unregistered Haitians. Roman Catholicism is the Haitian state religion, although there is also a sizable Protestant following. Voodoo, a synthesis of Catholicism and African tribal rituals, flourishes in rural Haiti and is practiced by many Haitian-Americans. A small number of Haitians practice magic or spiritual rituals, the details of which are not openly discussed by Haitians, especially to white foreigners.

## POTENTIAL RISK FACTORS FOR AIDS AMONG HAITIANS

Homosexuality is the major risk factor for 75% of AIDS patients in the United States. Epidemiologic data collected in Haiti reveals that almost all patients exhibit serologic evidence or histories of one or more sexually transmitted diseases, including syphilis, gonorrhea, and herpes simplex. As many as 20% of males with AIDS in Haiti admit to bisexuality.

For economic reasons, some Haitian men resort to prostitution, pandering to vacationing homosexuals, many of whom are from the United States. Carre-four, a suburb of Port-au-Prince, the Haitian capital, is the center of both male and female prostitution. It is probably no coincidence that Carre-four is also the epicenter of the AIDS epidemic in Haiti. Whereas 98% of the population lives in rural areas, fewer than 5% of the AIDS cases come from the countryside.

In a society that is so staunchly Catholic, and in which the macho image is avidly cultivated, the stigma of homosexuality is a formidable disincentive to candor in the discussion of sexual habits. Thus, it is likely that the prevalence of homosexuality in Haiti is underestimated. Heterosexual promiscuity by bisexual males may also explain the high incidence of AIDS among women in Haiti. In the United States, despite concerted efforts to elicit histories of homosexuality, fewer than 5% of Haitians will admit to such relationships at any time during their lives. Having distanced themselves from the economic climate that promoted homosexual prostitution, and having assumed a more conventional lifestyle in the United States, most are understandably reluctant to make such admissions. There is no evidence to implicate intravenous-narcotics abuse as an important means of transmission among Haitians. In addition to a cultural prohibition of such abuses, the cost of drugs and paraphernalia is prohibitive.

Because of the expense and scarcity of medical supplies, some physicians in Haiti may reuse needles and syringes without adequate sterilization, thus raising the specter of iatrogenic (physician-induced) transmission of disease. However, no such cases have been proven.

Many Haitians use potions and concoctions from herbs and roots (Harwood, 1979). The specific chemical constituents and their potential for immunosuppression are unknown. Antibiotics available over the counter are also sometimes used indiscriminately to treat various recurrent infections (Leonides and Hyppolite, 1983). Antibiotics may be immunosuppressive but, as with potions used for many years without apparent ill effects, are unlikely to be the primary cause of severe immune depression in these patients.

Animal sacrifice in voodoo rituals is occasionally accompanied by consumption of animal blood or uncooked meat by one or more of the participants (Metraux, 1958). Some investigators have speculated that the AIDS agent may be a variant or mutant form of an animal virus. Parvovirus and African swine fever virus are two such candidate agents, although there is no proof as yet to implicate either in AIDS. Were the AIDS agent indeed an animal virus, ritual practices might permit transmission from animal to man and, later, from person to person by other means. Magic ritual provides a means for transfer of blood and secretions from person to person. Women have been known to introduce menstrual blood into the food and drink of their partners to prevent them from "straying." Worshippers of Erzulie, a benign deity, engage in rituals during which the hougan, or priest, may engage in intercourse with other male worshippers. With our present level of ignorance about the prevalence and forms of Haitian rituals, one must consider any suggestion of disease transmission by ritual practices as purely speculative.

Transfusion-related cases of AIDS among Haitians have not been documented. In Haiti, 20% of patients questioned had had blood transfusions from 1½ to 6 years prior to the onset of disease (Pape et al., 1983). No reliable transfusion history is available for the majority of Haitian-Americans. Further study of this possible mode of transmission would be greater facilitated by the identification of a marker for AIDS that can be measured in the transfused unit of blood, as we now identify units contaminated with hepatitis B virus.

The antigenic-overload hypothesis suggests that a combination of factors (multiple viral, parasitic, bacterial, and fungal infections, and exposure to recreational and prescription drugs) contributes to a state of immune depression, eventually predisposing the patient to opportunistic infections and malignancy. As previously noted, venereal diseases and intestinal parasitic infections are common among Haitians in Haiti. Aside from the tendency of recurrent or chronic infections to produce a state of general debilitation, there is experimental evidence that the interaction of a patient's immune system with components of an infecting parasite may cause serious depression of cell-mediated immunity (Pearce, 1983). Antibodies directed against the parasite may cross-react with the host's own lymphocytes and render them dysfunctional. In addition, the parasite may produce substances that stimulate suppressor-cell activity or suppress helper-cell activity.

Poor sanitation and overcrowding in the cities of Haiti provide a favorable milieu for the spread of various infections from person to person or by insect vectors such as flies and mosquitos. These modes of transmission would not be expected to play an important role in the temperate climate of the United States.

Central Africa, and especially Zaire, has become a focus of attention after recent reports of AIDS or AIDS-like disease there dating back to 1976, several years prior to the onset of the epidemic in the Western Hemisphere. Equatorial Africa has been recognized for some time as an endemic region for KS, where it constitutes 9–12% of all malignancies. The recognition of opportunistic infections characteristic of AIDS has fostered speculation that the AIDS agent may have had its origin in Africa.

## IS BEING HAITIAN A RISK FACTOR FOR AIDS?

There is no evidence to implicate either a racial or ethnic predisposition to the development of AIDS. KS, the most common malignancy

afflicting homosexuals with AIDS, is associated with a specific genetic marker, the HLA-DR5 antigen, which can be detected on the
surfaces of the host's cells. About 65% of patients with KS have the
HLA-DR5 antigen, as compared to a frequency of only 12–20% in
the general population or in AIDS patients with opportunistic infections alone. This association suggests that cells carrying the HLA-
DR5 gene, or some closely related gene, are more susceptible to malignant change by an as yet unidentified stimulus. Interestingly, black
Africans have a higher prevalence of the HLA-DR5 antigen on their
cells (up to 50%) than do whites (Macek, 1982). There are as yet no
published genetic studies of Haitians with AIDS.

## SOCIAL AND ECONOMIC IMPACT OF AIDS

The original reports of AIDS among Haitian immigrants were sen-
sationalized and misrepresented in the popular press. Some news
broadcasts pictured scantily clad black natives dancing frenetically
about ritual fires, while others caricatured Haitians with AIDS as illegal aliens interned in detention camps. The fact that the majority of
Haitian AIDS victims fit neither of these stereotypes was ignored.
The impression left with the public in many instances was that AIDS
was pervasive throughout the Haitian community. Unlike the homosexual or drug addict, the Haitian was a highly visible victim of the
epidemic who could be singled out by virtue of his ethnic and cultural features.

Unfounded anxiety over the risks of acquiring AIDS by casual
contact resulted in widespread discrimination against Haitians in
housing and employment. Many were dismissed from their jobs,
while others were not given fair consideration for positions for which
they were qualified. Parents expressed fears that their children might
contract AIDS from Haitian domestics or from Haitian classmates in
school. The Haitian community responded with appropriate concern
for the health of its members and with understandable anger at what
they consider unfair and racist treatment. Dialogues between Haitian
and American physicians have helped to cool tempers and to educate
both the Haitian and non-Haitian communities about AIDS in general and about the scope of the problem among Haitian-Americans in
particular.

In response to political pressures brought to bear by representatives of the Haitian community, the New York City Department of Health has deleted "Haitian" as a risk group designation. Haitians with AIDS, but with no recognized risk factor such as homosexuality, drug abuse, or hemophilia, are included in the group designated "others." However, the CDC has thus far declined to eliminate the "Haitian" designation.

Limited resources are being increasingly taxed as more Haitian AIDS patients survive to return to the community. Many, lacking family support and unable to resume regular employment, need counseling and financial assistance. Haitian civic and religious groups are soliciting private and government funds to provide for the needs of AIDS victims, as well as for educational programs directed at the community at large.

Meanwhile, in Haiti, aside from the public health consequences of the disease, AIDS has had an impact on one of the major sources of Haiti's foreign exchange—tourism. In the aftermath of the reports of AIDS in Haitian-Americans, the tourist trade declined by 20%. Although the picture has recently improved somewhat, considerable anxiety is still expressed by travelers to Haiti.

### UNRAVELING THE MYSTERY

A multicenter case-control study of Haitian-Americans in Brooklyn, New York and in Miami, Florida and an independent case-control study in Haiti are in progress. As with the case-control study carried out by the CDC to investigate risk factors for AIDS among homosexuals, the design of these studies involves an extensive questionnaire. AIDS patients and control subjects, culled from clinic populations, private physician's offices, and hospitalized Haitians without AIDS, will be asked about such details as their past and present residences, occupations, sexual habits, ritual practices, transfusions, vaccination and infectious diseases history, and use of recreational and prescription drugs. Statistically significant differences between cases and controls may provide insights into the mechanisms of transmission of AIDS. For instance, if 60% of male Haitians with AIDS admit to bisexual activity compared to 5% of Haitian males of similar age but without AIDS, the implication would be that homosexual contact was an important risk factor for acquiring AIDS. Given the cultural and linguistic barriers cited above, it is possible that these surveys will be unable to define the risk factors for many, if not most, Haitians, particularly Haitian-Americans who may be unwilling to confide in non-Haitian interviewers.

## SUMMARY

The acquired immune deficiency syndrome (AIDS) is a new, lethal disease characterized by functional defects in the cell-mediated and humoral (antibody-forming) immune systems. It is manifested clinically by unusual malignancies and a variety of infections, especially those due to opportunistic pathogens.

It is hypothesized that the basic immune defect is triggered by an infection with an agent, most likely a virus, transmitted from person to person by blood or sexual contact. Unlike the other risk groups who have readily identifiable means of exposure to a putative AIDS agent, Haitians have posed an enigma until recently. Studies in Haiti have demonstrated that several aspects of Haitian lifestyle, not previously revealed in the questioning of Haitian-Americans, may provide mechanisms of transmission. Homosexual practices in particular appear to be significant for a sizable minority of patients. Transfusions, heterosexual promiscuity, contaminated needle exposure, and ritual practices may also play lesser roles.

Case-control studies being carried out with the cooperation of Haitian and American physicians will attempt to clarify the full spectrum of risk factors for Haitians with AIDS.

In the meantime, there is no reason to assume that Haitians as a group present a special public health risk.

# 9     Hemophiliacs, Blood Transfusions, and AIDS

## ROBERT HIRSCH

### CAN AIDS BE TRANSMITTED BY BLOOD: FEARS

Evidence available to date suggests that blood may play a role in the transmission of AIDS from one human being to another. As a result, a fear of all contact with blood has developed among both laymen and health-care workers. Some patients are reluctant to accept needed blood transfusions, others request blood only from family members or friends, some hospital and laboratory workers are afraid to give much needed personal care to patients or to perform laboratory tests of blood samples, and even some loyal donors have stopped giving blood.

These inappropriate reactions are in response to the serious nature of the disease and the frightening gaps in our knowledge of its diagnosis, treatment, and prevention. However, data are available to permit reasonable estimates of the risks involved. Moreover, it is possible to establish rational precautions to reduce risks for those exposed to blood, either accidentally or in the course of normal activities.

### CAN AIDS BE TRANSMITTED BY BLOOD: FACTS

#### Shared Needles—The Intravenous-Drug User

Seventeen percent of all AIDS patients are intravenous-drug users. This was the first information to indicate that AIDS might be transmitted by the passage of blood from one individual to another. People who inject themselves with habit-forming drugs often share needles without cleaning or sterilizing them between uses, enabling blood containing an agent that can cause disease to pass from person to person. Such transmission of hepatitis B, malaria, and other blood-borne infections have been well documented. Currently, it is assumed that AIDS in such drug users is also transmitted by this route rather than through any other shared characteristic.

### Blood Transfusions—Ten Million Pints Per Year

Blood-borne diseases can also be transmitted by blood transfusion. However, the risk of exposure is much lower than among drug users due to the care exercised in selecting healthy donors. Donors must be free of any symptoms or history of disease, and laboratory tests are done on all blood before it is distributed for transfusion.

More than 10 million pints of blood are collected per year in the United States. Much of it is subdivided into two or more component parts, such as red or white blood cells, platelets, and plasma. These components are usually transfused as units from a single donation, or as pools of 6 to 20 units in the case of platelets and leukocytes (white blood cells). A small number of patients may receive several hundred products per year, but the average patient receives only 3 units. From mid-1981 to mid-1984, about 45 million blood components were transfused, but only 52 cases of AIDS were verified in recipients who were not members of recognized high-risk groups. Assuming that blood was the transmitter of AIDS in these cases, the risk of contracting AIDS is about one in a million. This is far less than the chance of developing hepatitis; it is estimated that 10% of transfused patients develop some form of hepatitis, often not serious enough to produce symptoms.

In addition to over 500 reported cases of transfusion-related hepatitis per year in the United States, 9 cases of malaria were transmitted by blood transfusion in 1982. These adverse results must be weighed against the benefits derived from a blood transfusion. For example, they keep bleeding patients alive, permit operations that entail heavy blood loss as an unavoidable part of the procedure, and maintain normal blood counts in patients with incurable anemia. It is obvious that such benefits far outweigh the small risk, even of a disease as serious as AIDS.

If blood transfusions can transmit AIDS, then one would expect to find AIDS in both blood donors and recipients. AIDS, in common with other contagious diseases such as syphilis and hepatitis, must be reported to the public health authorities by the patient's physician. The CDC combed these reports for donor-recipient pairs who developed AIDS. In 1984, the CDC reported details of 7 cases of AIDS among blood recipients. These patients, who were not in any of the recognized high-risk groups, had received between 2 and 48 transfusions of blood or blood components within 5 years of developing AIDS. In every case, at least one high-risk donor was found. None had full-blown AIDS, but several had abnormal laboratory tests or enlarged lymph nodes. The report concluded that these findings strengthened, but did not necessarily prove, the supposition that AIDS may be transmitted by blood.

### Blood Coagulation Products—Treatment of Hemophilia

Plasma, the liquid portion of blood, contains various proteins useful in treating patients. As a first step in the separation and purification of these proteins, plasma from many donors is pooled. Treatment with any one of these products may involve material from many donors. Hemophiliac patients, for example, may receive one type of blood product (cryoprecipitate) prepared from 6–12 donors, or another (Factor-VIII concentrate) prepared from a pool of plasma from 2,500–10,000 donors. Both types of treatment are given many times per year, either to stop a bleeding episode or to prevent new ones. Thus, a hemophiliac is exposed to thousands of blood donors per year, in contrast to the average blood recipient who is exposed to only 3 per year.

Because the effective protein in both cryoprecipitate and Factor VIII is easily destroyed by heat, they cannot be sterilized at high temperatures. Thus, the hemophiliac is exposed to any viruses present in the original pool. As a result, many more hemophiliacs have contracted hepatitis from blood coagulation products than have patients receiving blood products from single donors. On the basis of this information, researchers have been looking for cases of AIDS among hemophiliacs who are not members of any of the high-risk groups.

To date, no hemophiliac receiving cryoprecipitate has developed AIDS, but 37 receiving Factor-VIII concentrate have done so. It would appear that pooling plasma from large numbers of donors may make Factor-VIII concentrate capable of transmitting AIDS. However, a note of caution is necessary in interpreting these data. Each pool of plasma yields enough Factor VIII to treat up to 100 patients. If a pool is contaminated by an agent that can cause AIDS, then most, if not all, of the 100 patients served by that pool might be expected to develop AIDS. This has not happened. Fourteen of the 16 hemophiliacs who developed AIDS each received a different batch of Factor VIII; only one pair of patients shared the same batch. This finding suggests that either patients differ in susceptibility to AIDS, and only 1 or 2 of 100 exposed people contract the disease, or Factor-VIII concentrate is not the source of the disease.

**Serum Albumin—The Lesson of Pasteurization**

Two other blood products are prepared from large pools of plasma: serum albumin and gamma globulin. The former is not sensitive to moderate heat and is routinely pasteurized at 60°C for 10 hours, which kills most known viruses. No case of a known viral or other infectious disease has been reported in patients receiving albumin exclusively, nor has AIDS developed in any albumin recipient who was not a member of a recognized high-risk group. These facts suggest, but do not prove, that AIDS may be caused by an agent that is destroyed by pasteurization.

As a result of these findings, a search is on to find a way to treat Factor-VIII concentrates that destroys all viruses without altering Factor VIII. Two approaches are under investigation. One is an attempt to find a combination of temperature and time that kills viruses but does not destroy Factor VIII. The other is an attempt to find chemicals that accomplish the same end and that are easily removed from the final product. Both procedures use the hepatitis B virus as the test marker, since the causative agent of AIDS is not known conclusively. No completely safe and effective method has yet been found.

**Gamma Globulin—A Safe Product**

Gamma globulin contains the antibodies produced by the donor's body to guard against infections. The antibodies develop when a person either recovers from a disease, such as measles or hepatitis, or receives a vaccine to develop immunity against a specific disease. No gamma-globulin recipient has been reported to have contracted any disease, including AIDS, even though gamma globulin cannot be pasteurized. Just why this is true is not known. It is thought that, because gamma globulin is made from a pool of plasma from so many different donors, it probably contains antibodies to all known viruses. These antibodies combine with and inactivate the viruses, rendering them noninfectious. By implication then, if AIDS also is caused by an infectious agent such as a virus, there may be antibodies to AIDS. This is encouraging, because it means that if and when such an infectious agent is found, a vaccine may be developed that will protect everyone from getting AIDS.

**Hepatitis-B Immune Globulin and Hepatitis-B Vaccine—Risks versus Benefits**

The fear that AIDS is an infectious disease communicable by blood products has created a problem with respect to two products recently developed to combat hepatitis B infections: hepatitis B immune globulin (HBIG) and hepatitis B vaccine. HBIG is gamma globulin made from pools of plasma from donors who have had hepatitis B and developed a high concentration of antibodies against the virus. It is given to people accidentally exposed to hepatitis B by a finger-stick with a needle or glass tube contaminated with blood containing the virus. HBIG confers temporary protection and prevents the infection from developing.

Hepatitis B vaccine is prepared from plasma containing the virus itself, treated to kill the virus, and is obtained from donors who are carriers of hepatitis B. The treatment prevents the virus from causing the disease, but those injected with the vaccine still produce antibodies against the virus. Vaccination imparts a lifelong protection against hepatitis B.

The major source of plasma containing hepatitis antibodies and live hepatitis B virus has been male homosexual donors. Because the source is a high-risk group for AIDS, people have become reluctant to use these products. However, since no variety of gamma globulin has been associated with AIDS, the risk must be considered small or nonexistent. The benefit of preventing hepatitis B infection, which sometimes results in chronic illness or death, far outweighs the risk.

Since the treatment to kill the hepatitis B virus in the vaccine has been shown to be effective enough to kill all known viruses, it bears repeating that the opportunity to protect against the disease, especially in health-care workers who are constantly exposed to hepatitis B, warrants the minimal risk.

## REDUCING THE RISK OF TRANSMITTING AIDS VIA BLOOD TRANSFUSION

The transmission of AIDS by blood transfusion has not been proven. Nevertheless, due to the serious nature of the disease, blood collecting agencies in the United States have assumed that it may be transmitted by blood and have adopted procedures to reduce the risk.

### Screening of Donors

Potential blood donors have always been carefully screened to eliminate anyone who is not in excellent health. Donors are made aware of the general criteria in advance and are then carefully questioned by a health professional at the blood collection site. The questions deal with the history of past diseases and symptoms of current ailments. Also, blood pressure, pulse, temperature, and blood hemoglobin level are measured. This system has been in place for many years and works very well. Volunteer donors can be relied on to answer health questions truthfully, and the blood supply derived from them is remarkably safe.

As information about AIDS accumulated, it became apparent that additional steps were needed in the screening procedure. These were designed to notify people in groups at increased risk of exposure to AIDS that they should not donate, as well as to check for symptoms known to be associated with the disease. Brochures and letters listed the high-risk groups and explained that even healthy individuals in these groups might be AIDS carriers. In the health screening examination, donors were now questioned about unexplained weight loss, prolonged fever, persistent cough or diarrhea, night sweats, enlarged lymph nodes, or bruise-like spots on the skin that did not go away. None of these symptoms is exclusive to AIDS, since any one or more may be a consequence of other ailments. However, since no test is yet known to distinguish between AIDS and other causes of these symptoms, it seems wise to postpone blood donation until the symptoms disappear.

A special problem exists in the screening of donors for AIDS. For personal reasons, members of high-risk groups may be extremely reluctant to acknowledge that they are in the high-risk category. Thus, it is very important that the health screening process be carried out privately. However, even this may not give sufficient assurance of confidentiality, and a suspicious donor may be tempted to give false information. Consequently, a safeguard was added, consisting of having the donor indicate whether or not the donated unit should be used for transfusion (rather than for research or other purposes), using a form that bears the unit identification number but no name. The donor donates and leaves. The donated unit is later removed from inventory at a remote station where the donor cannot be identified. Studies of the effectiveness of these steps at one large regional blood center indicated that the combination of informational brochures, additional health questions, and confidential exclusion of units is working effectively to reduce any possible risk of transmitting AIDS by blood transfusions.

### Autologous Blood Transfusion—Donating for One's Own Use

Fear of contracting AIDS has renewed interest in a procedure for providing blood for oneself (autologous: derived from the same person). People in otherwise good health who are scheduled for a surgical procedure donate a unit of their own blood in advance, to be placed on reserve for use at the time of the operation. It is even possible to arrange for advance collection of up to 3 or 4 pints of blood. This procedure relies on a complex process of collecting a unit and later returning it to the donor. While this technique reduces the risk of exposure to most hazards associated with blood transfusions, it is useful only when the individual is healthy, is not anemic, and has enough time to make the arrangements. Most people who need blood transfusions are not in this category. A further disadvantage to this technique is that it requires complex clerical procedures that significantly increase the risk of error in blood transfusion therapy. There is no room for errors. Since red cells can be frozen and stored for several years, it is theoretically possible for people to donate blood while they are healthy and have it stored in a freezer until needed.

However, this is completely impractical because it would require vast storehouses for frozen blood, some of which would never be used.

**The Fallacy of the Dedicated Donor**

Another way people try to protect themselves against AIDS is to use a "dedicated donor." Such a donor is recruited from among relatives and friends, in the belief that known or related donors are necessarily safer than strangers. The three major U.S. blood bank organizations—the Council of Community Blood Banks, the American National Red Cross, and the American Association of Blood Banks—have issued a joint statement pointing out the fallacy of such reasoning and agreeing on a policy to oppose this practice.

The main reason for not accepting dedicated donors is that they often are too dedicated. On the one hand, friends or relatives may not be acceptable as blood donors because they are not in good health, have been exposed to communicable diseases, or have a disease they do not want to divulge. On the other hand, they are so concerned about the welfare of their relative or friend who requires a blood transfusion that, consciously or not, they may not answer the health-history questions truthfully. In an effort to do good, they may actually do harm. The safest donor is the true volunteer who gains no advantage from donating—neither money, special privileges, days off, nor the chance to do someone a favor.

A second important reason for not earmarking specific donations for specific patients is that this adds extra procedures to the collecting, testing, and distributing of blood. Each additional step increases the risk of error.

## THE SEARCH FOR A BLOOD TEST FOR AIDS

An extensive search is being made for a blood test that would indicate whether or not a person has AIDS or blood containing an agent that might transmit AIDS to someone else. Three different approaches are being followed. The first is a search for an infectious agent, such as a virus or bacteria, that might be the cause of AIDS. Early studies found that AIDS patients often show evidence of a past or present infection by the Epstein-Barr virus, which causes infectious mononucleosis. Another virus possibly associated with AIDS is cytomegalovirus, which causes disease in newborn infants and immunosuppressed individuals. However, healthy people also show evidence of carrying these viruses, and no definitive link has been demonstrated between either virus and AIDS.

More recently, an association has been noted between AIDS and a family of retroviruses. The first in this family was discovered in patients infected with human T-cell leukemia virus (HTLV-I). A second member of the family, HTLV-II, appears to be associated with a variant of this leukemia. Two research groups, operating independently, have now isolated a third member of this family, called HTLV-III, from the T cells of patients with AIDS, from patients with diffuse, persistent lymph-node enlargement (thought by some to be a pre-AIDS condition), and from a few patients in high-risk groups but without overt AIDS. (Actually, one of the research groups, in the United States, isolated HTLV-III. The other, in France, isolated the lymphadenopathy virus, LAV. Evidence strongly suggests that the two are really the same, single virus.)

In one donor-recipient pair, HTLV-III was isolated from both the high-risk donor, who developed AIDS long after having donated the blood, and the recipient, who developed AIDS 7 months after the transfusion. The recipient was not a member of any of the high-risk groups.

These new developments strongly suggest a cause-and-effect relationship between HTLV-III and AIDS. A major effort is now under way to develop a simple laboratory technique to mass screen blood samples for the presence of HTLV-III particles or their antibodies.

The second approach to a possible test for AIDS involves studies of the immune system. Underlying AIDS is a suppression of the immune system's ability to recognize and eliminate foreign material, such as bacteria, viruses, parasites, and pollens. Tests that show abnormal immune functions would suggest that the patient has AIDS, even without other signs of illness. Two important indications of the health of the immune system are the total number of lymphocytes (one form of white blood cells) circulating in the blood and the ratio between the numbers of T-helper and T-suppressor lymphocytes. A low total lymphocyte count and a low ratio of T-helper/T-suppressor cells are seen in almost all AIDS patients, and members of high-risk groups tend to have lymphocyte counts intermediate between healthy people and AIDS patients. However, since various other diseases show the same abnormalities, this test is not conclusively diagnostic of AIDS. Other tests of the immune system are also being evaluated.

The third approach is a search for tests that detect so-called surrogate markers of AIDS. Surrogate markers are substances that may have nothing directly to do with AIDS, but whose blood levels may change as a direct or indirect result of AIDS. One such marker is a protein known as beta-2 microglobulin found on the surface of many cells, including lymphocytes. A very small amount is normally present in plasma, probably as a product of the normal destruction of old lymphocytes. In AIDS patients, the concentration is increased, possibly due to an increased rate of lymphocyte destruction. However, since other diseases may produce the same effect, this test also is not a reliable indicator of AIDS.

## THE SAFETY OF DONATING BLOOD

A recent public opinion poll by the Roper Agency reported that 91% of all Americans know about AIDS, about 50% think they can get AIDS from receiving blood transfusions, and 26% believe they can get AIDS from donating blood. The belief in donor risks is a total misconception.

One simply cannot get AIDS by donating blood. There are no AIDS patients at the donation site; all who are present are in the best of health. Personnel who collect the blood have been specially trained in techniques to prevent the spread of disease, and equipment used to draw blood is almost entirely disposable, that is, delivered in sealed, sterile containers, used once, and then discarded under rigorously sanitary conditions. Needles inserted into donors' veins are cut off from the tubing after use and placed in strong, covered containers to prevent handlers or others from being stuck by a used needle. On the rare occasion that blood is spilled or gets into a nondisposable instrument, it is immediately removed with solutions that thoroughly disinfect the area.

The best evidence of safety is the record of the nursing staff. Collectively, this group has been exposed to tens of millions of blood donors and their donations, and not one case of AIDS has been reported among them. The strict hygenic measures used for many years by blood collection facilities have completely protected donors and staff. Without a doubt, giving blood is safe.

## SUMMARY

The principal reasons for suspecting that AIDS can be transmitted from one human to another by blood transfusion are:

Seventeen percent of all AIDS patients are intravenous-drug users who often share needles without cleaning or sterilizing them.

A small number of people who receive transfusions of blood or blood products, such as Factor-VIII concentrates, but who are not in any of the high-risk groups, have developed AIDS.

In a group of 7 blood recipients who developed AIDS, at least one donor for each recipient was found to be a member of a high-risk group.

HTLV-III was isolated from both members of a donor-recipient pair who both developed AIDS.

The risk of developing AIDS from transfusions appears to be less than one in a million. The risk in hemophiliacs appears to be higher, probably because they receive repeated injections of Factor VIII, a blood coagulation factor prepared from pools of plasma from 2,500 to 10,000 donors. Nevertheless, only a very small number of hemophiliacs have developed AIDS. No AIDS has been associated with serum albumin or gamma globulin, two other plasma proteins prepared from large pools, probably because the former is pasteurized and the latter contains a rich pool of antibodies.

Careful screening of donors has been instituted to eliminate members of high AIDS-risk groups. Strict confidentiality protects the donor's privacy. Autologous blood transfusion, where possible and practical, also reduces the risk of transmitting AIDS. Dedicated donors, chosen by recipients to donate blood for use only for the recipients themselves, are not considered as safe as anonymous, volunteer donors who are more likely to answer the health-screening questions fully and honestly.

Procedures are being developed to identify blood products that might transmit AIDS. They are intended to detect HTLV-III virus particles or their antibodies in the blood; reveal deficiencies in a potential donor's immune system; or indicate surrogate markers for AIDS, substances in blood that may have nothing directly to do with AIDS, but increase or decrease as a secondary consequence of AIDS.

AIDS cannot be contracted by donating blood. All pieces of equipment, including needles, are new, used once, and thrown away. Strict hygienic measures used by all blood collection agencies completely protect the donor against disease.

# 10    Is the General Public at Risk?

### ARYE RUBINSTEIN

## A RATIONAL PERSPECTIVE

Is there a danger of AIDS spreading to the general public? This is the main question that torments the scientific community, the mass media, and the general public. AIDS is undoubtedly a major public health issue, but not of the magnitude of a plague. As with many epidemics of the past, the best response to ignorance and misinformation concerning AIDS is scientific reasoning. Whether or not the human T-cell leukemia virus HTLV-III or the lymphadenopathy virus LAV (which may both be the same single virus) proves to be the deadly causative agent, a fairly reliable concept of the epidemiology of the disease has been developed through the analysis of AIDS transmission in the major cohorts at high risk.

Who are the major risk groups for AIDS? The first and most studied group is homosexual and bisexual males, who comprise about 72–77% of all AIDS patients. Only rarely is AIDS acquired by female sexual partners of AIDS patients. The second largest group (about 15%) includes intravenous-drug users. In both major groups, the risk factors are well recognized. For example, avoidance of sexual contact with AIDS patients, restriction of homosexual activities to a limited number of partners, and refrainment from needle sharing can theoretically control the contagion of the disease among homosexuals and drug users.

Women were initially thought to be excluded from risk groups. In fact, it was stated that lesbians are free of AIDS and may thus be an ideal blood-donor population. The emergence of AIDS among women was, nevertheless, not a surprise to AIDS experts. Women acquired the disease as frequently as men from the use of intravenous drugs and, more rarely, through sexual contact with males who belonged to one of the high-risk groups. The fear of a major AIDS epidemic was revived when the disease also developed in other patient populations, such as recipients of blood and blood products, recent Haitian immigrants, children of members of high-risk populations, and individuals outside of any recognized risk group.

A close look at these new patient populations does not, however, justify the fears. On the contrary, scientific analysis of these patients should alleviate anxiety about a possible epidemic. In this chapter, relevant epidemiologic aspects of various patient populations will be addressed, and then the focus will be on lessons learned from the study of children with AIDS and of their families, including siblings of infant AIDS victims. These lessons provide a model for predicting the potential spread of the disease.

## EPIDEMIOLOGY

The number of AIDS patients who do not belong to the two major groups at risk comprise no more than 6% of the total, a percentage that has remained constant as more data have accumulated. If AIDS agent(s) had contaminated blood supplies in the United States, or if the disease were highly contagious, a much larger number of AIDS victims would have been expected. Moreover, the risk of acquiring AIDS in the United States through transfusions of blood or blood products was calculated to be 1 or 2 per million transfusions. This is extremely low compared to risks of other transfusion reactions. The experience abroad has been similar. For example, in Japan, where about two-thirds of administered blood or blood products is derived from American donors, no AIDS due to blood transfusions has been detected to date.

Theoretically, the patients most likely to acquire AIDS from blood products are recipients of multiple transfusions and those whose immunity is suppressed, e.g., cancer patients and recipients of kidney transplants. (Transplant patients are given potent drugs that destroy their immunity to prevent rejection of the alien tissues. Cancer patients similarly receive chemotherapy that renders them immunodeficient.) These patients frequently receive multiple transfusions and yet none, except hemophiliacs, have contracted AIDS. Even among hemophiliacs, the number of AIDS victims is so small that some investigators are reluctant to use this incidence to link blood transfusions and AIDS.

It has been postulated that the epidemiology of AIDS mimics that of hepatitis B, since both diseases are transmitted by needle sticks, blood transfusions, and sexual contact. However, infection with hepatitis B is quite ubiquitous while AIDS is relatively rare. If AIDS is really transmitted along the hepatitis routes, then the number of AIDS patients should be 10 or 100 times greater than it is, unless the AIDS agent is of extremely low infectivity. Moreover, although health-care workers are frequently exposed to hepatitis B, AIDS has not been reported among them.

Several medical centers have been studying health-care personnel who have had close contact with AIDS patients, particularly those who have inadvertently been stuck with a needle used for an AIDS patient or were otherwise exposed to AIDS blood, e.g., through a skin abrasion. In most medical centers, the exposure of health-care personnel to AIDS patients was not controlled by meaningful precautionary measures until late 1982. Blood was often drawn without gloves, AIDS patients' secretions were not specially handled, and blood-count samples were spread thinly on glass slides without protection. Moreover, many patients received surgical procedures or were bronchoscoped before it was known that they had AIDS. During bronchoscopy, the lungs are examined through a tube passed down the airways, and the examiner is exposed to secretions and blood coughed up by the patient. If AIDS behaved like a highly infectious disease, these health-care workers should have been likely victims. However, only 4 health-care workers, not apparent members of recognized high-risk groups, have so far contracted the disease.

These 4 cases aroused a near panic among health-care workers, which subsided when the cases were analyzed statistically. Such analysis requires an estimate of how many cases might have been expected merely on the basis of chance. Such a calculation was reported by Dr. R. S. Gordon of the National Institutes of Health.

In mid-July 1983, the total number of AIDS cases that had been reported to the Centers for Disease Control (CDC) was 1902, of whom 110 could not be assigned to any designated high-risk groups. Four health workers were among the 110. According to the 1980 census, the United States population of ages 18–64 totaled 137.2 million. This age span encompasses almost all employed persons and virtually all AIDS cases. The National Center for Health Statistics reports that in 1980 approximately 7.23 million persons were employed in the health industry. If employment in the health industry bears no relationship to the risk of AIDS, then the number of health workers expected among the 100 "unexplained" AIDS cases = 110 × 7.23/137.2 = 5.8, which exceeds the 4 cases observed. No elaborate statistical analysis is required to demonstrate that this comparison refutes the hypothesis that health workers are at increased risk for AIDS. On the other hand, neither does it argue for cavalier disregard of prudent precautions. Encouragingly, our recent studies in collaboration with the CDC have so far shown no antibody titers to LAV-1 in sera from health-care workers who had prolonged and intensive contact with AIDS patients.

## AIDS IN CHILDREN

Perhaps most fascinating and perplexing is the epidemiologic significance of AIDS in children. In 1979, we encountered a child with recurrent infections suggestive of an immunodeficiency. However, this child's immunologic work-up revealed abnormalities different from any known congenital immunodeficiencies (inborn defects of the immune system). The child also presented with the unusual findings of markedly enlarged lymph nodes and swelling of the salivary glands. The most provocative discovery was that the child's mother had the same symptoms and the same immunodeficiency.

In 1981, when AIDS was reported in adults, we realized that this child and his mother had AIDS. Since 1981, the number of infants we have seen with AIDS has increased sharply. By June 1982, we had treated 7 such infants, by January 1983 the number was 13, and at present 65 children with AIDS are followed in our clinic.

As with all other newly discovered patient populations at risk for AIDS, the disease in children soon reached the headlines of the news media, and a new wave of alarm was created. When we and others found families with more than 1 affected child, the level of anxiety rose even higher. "Here is the proof for the spread of AIDS to the general population," "AIDS may spread from child to child by casual contact" were typical of the fearful statements expressed by the public. These fears derived from the perplexing question of how these infants acquired the disease.

It took us several months to resolve this question. Our medical center is located in a geographic area where AIDS leaped to epidemic proportions among intravenous-drug abusers. The mothers of all infants with AIDS, except for one, admitted to intravenous-drug abuse. When these women were examined, many were found to have an immunodeficiency identical to that of their infants. Moreover, with time, several developed the clinical symptoms characteristic of AIDS and 6 died. These findings clearly linked the disease in children to that in their mothers.

When did the children acquire AIDS from their mothers? Retrospective analysis suggested that the mean age of onset of clinical disease was 5 to 6 months. In adults, the incubation period for AIDS is estimated to be between 6 and 33 months. The general rule is that incubation periods of infections are shorter in immunodeficient patients, who are incapable of preventing the penetration of body surfaces by microorganisms and often are unable to inhibit the reproduction of or destroy the invading pathogen. As a result of these deficiencies in the host, the organisms have free access to the body and multiply much faster.

Newborns are physiologically immunodeficient and more prone to acquire various infections. Thus, a shorter incubation period, probably a few months, for the AIDS agent could be expected in young infants. Since the disease in infants started in the first months of life, we suspected that AIDS could have been acquired *in utero* (in the womb) or shortly after birth. During birth, the newborn has ample contact with maternal blood and can acquire AIDS via blood as do hemophiliacs and intravenous-drug users. If, however, the disease is acquired in the womb, the AIDS agent must be capable of penetrating the placenta. For a long time we were unable to determine definitively if the children acquired the disease before, during, or after birth. As time passed, new facts shed light on this enigma.

Some infants with AIDS never left the nursery or were placed in foster care shortly after birth. Contact with their mothers was limited to the first days of life. We studied the foster parents and found them to be immunologically competent and healthy. However, the natural mothers of the babies with AIDS were found to have symptoms suggestive of AIDS and/or were immunodeficient. These circumstances strengthened our conviction that AIDS was transmitted to the babies in the womb or during birth.

Another interesting observation, in a family of intravenous-drug users, strengthened this hypothesis. Early in 1984, we diagnosed AIDS in a 22-month old child born to an intravenous-drug-using prostitute. The mother was pregnant again when we first studied her. When her baby was born, we watched carefully for symptoms of AIDS. The baby's psychomotor development appeared abnormal from birth and, within 2 weeks, the first bacterial infections were noted, followed at 4 months by fungal sepsis and meningitis.

Although the immunologic competence tested soon after birth was like that of a normal newborn, the fact that the infant's older brother had AIDS made us cautious and suspicious that the disease in the newborn was also AIDS and that an immunodeficiency might develop at any time. The fungus infection at 4 months was a bad omen. Soon after that infection, laboratory studies showed a progressive deterioration of the immunologic system until a pattern similar to that of the mother and older brother was reached. It was clear that the baby could not have acquired the disease from his brother since there had been no contact between them. Did the baby acquire the disease at birth or *in utero*? If he acquired it at birth, then the incubation period had to be only a few days or at most 2–3 weeks. This is an unreasonably short incubation period, inconsistent with all previous studies of adults with AIDS.

Therefore, the most likely hypothesis is that the AIDS agent infected the fetus in the womb. It is recognized that infections of the fetus (congenital infections) may damage various organs such as the brain and the heart. For example, babies with a congenital cytomegalovirus infection often have a microcephalus (small head), eye abnormalities, and retardation in development. Babies infected in the womb by *Toxoplasmosis gondii* (a parasite) may have a hydrocephalus (large, water-head), eye abnormalities, and large liver, spleen, and lymph nodes. Also, about 20 years ago, before rubella vaccine became available, infants in several countries were plagued by the congenital rubella syndrome. These babies were often severely retarded and had multiple organ abnormalities as a result of infection with the rubella virus *in utero* from their mothers. We have looked in vain for these congenital infections in AIDS babies. Yet, when we analyzed the abnormalities encountered in congenital infections, we found some immunologic similarities to AIDS. Many AIDS babies had a birth weight and length far too low for their gestational age, as is seen also in congenital infections. Also, many AIDS babies did not exhibit normal psychomotor development from birth, indicating damage to the brain *in utero*.

This information slightly allayed anxiety concerning the risk of AIDS to the general public. However, as in many earlier instances, a new controversy soon developed, this time over the finding that some families had more than one child with AIDS. We attempted to calm the public by suggesting that a second and third child may also have acquired the disease from the mother *in utero*. This hypothesis was rightly disputed by other scientists who argued that a mother who acquires an infectious disease during one pregnancy seldom transmits it to her children delivered in later pregnancies. For example, if a women has one baby with congenital toxoplasmosis, she is highly unlikely to have another baby with toxoplasmosis in her next pregnancy. This also applies to the congenital rubella syndrome. Once a woman has the disease, she develops immunity. The invading microorganisms are destroyed and the immunity prevents reinfection by the same microorganisms. If this is true, then of 2 siblings with AIDS only 1 acquired it *in utero* while the other may have acquired it by contact with the sick sibling. The latter possibility was further supported by the recent isolation of HTLV-III from the saliva of AIDS victims and healthy homosexual men.

This raises the possibility that the general population may acquire AIDS by intimate, but nonsexual, contact with AIDS patients. When our social workers and nurses visited the homes of children with AIDS, they were impressed by the unusually close contact between family members. In general, children with AIDS were born to families of low socioeconomic background who lived under poor hygienic conditions. The mother and several children often lived in one room. The child with AIDS was not toilet trained and often shared utensils or a bed with siblings. This was not casual contact, but an extremely intimate physical closeness that could facilitate the transmission of the disease in the family. Did one sibling transmit the disease to another? We were reluctant, for the reasons explained below, to accept the theory of intrafamilial spread via intimate contact.

Mothers of children with AIDS turned out to be almost uniformly immunodeficient. An immunodeficient individual will not develop proper immunity to an infecting organism and may be reinfected several times or carry the organism in the body for years, even a lifetime. Therefore, several children of an immunodeficient mother may acquire the same disease in consecutive pregnancies, and previous experience with rubella and toxoplasmosis in normal pregnant women does not apply to pregnant women who have AIDS.

We analyzed longitudinally the families that had more than one child with AIDS. When a second or third child of a family with an index patient developed AIDS, it was always a younger, never an older, sibling, suggesting transmission of AIDS *in utero*. Moreover, we studied the members of over a hundred households of AIDS patients for clinical or immunologic signs of AIDS. During a period of up to 4 years, no foster parents, older children in the family, or unrelated playmates of children with AIDS developed AIDS. Also, none showed evidence of serum antibodies to HTLV-III (or LAV).

These findings strongly supported our view that AIDS is not spread by intrafamilial association, even by intimate contact between children. Thus, the risk to the general population can be considered negligible.

If a mother transmits the disease to her offspring *in utero*, can we predict which mother is carrying the infection? What can we learn from these mothers about other carriers of AIDS? To answer this question, we studied the immunologic systems of all available mothers of AIDS infants. As mentioned earlier, most of these women were intravenous-drug users and most were immunodeficient and/or had clinical AIDS. One exception will be described in more detail.

The index patient in this family was a 16-month-old girl with AIDS. Unexpectedly, her mother was completely healthy and had no immunodeficiency. The father was an intravenous-drug user who also was healthy, but his blood revealed an immunodeficiency suggestive of AIDS. Did this infant acquire the disease postnatally from her father? If so, then the question of transmission by close contact between father and infant had to be reconsidered. The enigma was resolved, in part, when the mother gave birth to another infant, who was studied from birth. This newborn was found to be immunodeficient and thus must have acquired the disease *in utero*. With time, the mother's immune system also deteriorated in the direction of the classical AIDS profile.

These events indicate that both siblings possibly acquired the disease *in utero* from their mother. However, a missing link was the fact that the mother was healthy and immunocompetent at the time of delivery. Can a "healthy" mother carry the AIDS agent and transmit it to her offspring *in utero*? We believe so, although conclusive evidence still has to be brought forth. It is known from epidemiologic studies that many individuals develop immunity to a virus without exhibiting clinical disease. For example, many women have immunity to rubella without having had clinical disease in the past. Some individuals acquire a rubella infection without having even the slightest fever, malaise, or skin rash, and yet they were infected; their immune system recognizes the virus and provides a lifelong immunity.

Theoretically, the same may apply to the AIDS agent. We believe that many of us have encountered this agent and developed immunity to it without having any overt illness. Thus, healthy carriers of AIDS may be much more frequent than AIDS patients, and carriers may transmit the disease during pregnancy, via a needle stick, or through sexual contact.

These characteristics were previously observed in immunologic studies of hepatitis B, a virus that has been clearly identified. Similar immunologic tools to study the epidemiology of AIDS became available with the identification of HTLV-III/LAV-I. In fact, some mothers whose children have AIDS were found to have antibodies to these viruses but were clinically healthy, and thus qualify as the proposed healthy carriers of AIDS. The same may apply to healthy homosexual men at risk for AIDS in whom HTLV-III was found in semen, saliva, and blood cultures.

As happens with every infectious disease, one should expect that some cases of AIDS will be discovered for which no risk factors can be documented or are admitted by the patients. Such isolated cases should not refuel the fear of a general AIDS epidemic. Rather they should strengthen our conviction that AIDS will not spread to the general population and that, with the taking of necessary precautions, the incidence of AIDS will decline.

# 11     Ethical Issues in AIDS
## THOMAS H. MURRAY

To understand the ethical issues posed by AIDS, we must see it as a contravention of the general trend in modern medicine. It is an anachronism. In a society and a medical profession grown accustomed to the idea that the fight against disease is being progressively won, the appearance of a virulent new disease is an astonishment.

In this century, medicine has moved from being capable of providing only care and comfort to administering cures, beginning with the availability in the 1940s of penicillin and other antibiotics. Until that time, bacterial pneumonia and other infections were often lethal and the weapons of medicine were defenseless. Suddenly, physicians acquired the capacity to treat those infections and often to defeat death itself. Also, refinements in the skills of curing have mingled with the start of a new era—the era of control. We can, and at times literally do, control the functioning of organ systems. The respirator, which does the breathing when the lung and its muscles cannot, and the artificial kidney are two of the most common examples of twentieth-century mastery over death. It is now virtually possible to keep vital functions operating in the body of what was once a living person, and physicians have been known to refer to the practice of maintaining someone whose brain has ceased to function as "ventilating a corpse."

These dramatic and newly acquired abilities to cure and control bring in their wake great ethical dilemmas to which physicians and ethicists must direct their attention. The moral problems created by AIDS for the most part escape familiar categories, compel us to remember the earlier days of medicine, and require us to meld old problems with new understandings. The root of most contemporary dilemmas in medical ethics is the power conferred by our abilities to cure and control; in the case of AIDS almost the opposite is true. In AIDS, it is our powerlessness and ignorance that create the most difficult moral problems.

The ethical aspects of AIDS may be organized into four categories:

Moral responsibilities of health professionals
Moral responsibilities of researchers
Moral responsibilities of people with AIDS
Moral responsibilities of society

## MORAL RESPONSIBILITIES OF HEALTH PROFESSIONALS

Among physicians and nurses today, few remember that in the era of care and compassion, before the discovery of antibiotics, medicine and nursing were often dangerous professions. With the process of disease and contagion poorly understood and no effective treatment available for infection, those who cared for the sick risked illness themselves.

Though the time of greatest danger is past, hospitals are still one of the most dangerous work environments, principally due to the hazards of anesthetic and sterilizing gases and the chance of infection. These risks are usually regarded as routine and barely noticed. The fear inspired in some physicians and nurses by the advent of AIDS is therefore all the more surprising.

It must be said that there is no reliable information on the number of doctors and nurses who have refused to care for AIDS patients. In all likelihood, the vast majority of health professionals have behaved appropriately and accepted their responsibility to care for these patients. Still, the publicized cases of refusal, and the experiences and impressions of AIDS patients and of professional colleagues, indicate that some doctors and nurses have failed to show the courage and dedication we have come to expect of them. Dr. Joseph Sonnabend, a physician and researcher treating AIDS patients in New York City, bemoans the fear AIDS has inspired among health professionals: "All down the line there are frightened people. There are doctors and nurses refusing to treat sick people. I don't know why they went into the field in the first place" (Weiss, 1983).

Documented examples are less common. There have been reports of two nurses in Santa Clara, California who resigned rather than care for patients with AIDS (Weiss, 1983). Also, there is the sad case of Morgan McDonald. McDonald was an AIDS patient in a hospital in Gainesville, Florida. The hospital discharged him and arranged for him to be flown by chartered jet to San Francisco, where he was quickly admitted to San Francisco General Hospital. Mervyn Silverman, Director of Public Health for San Francisco, has quoted parts of a letter written by an attorney for the Gainesville Hospital, which said, among other things: "The attending physician has determined you're no longer in need of acute hospital care; that you're utilizing hospital space and resources that should otherwise be available to acutely ill patients." The hospital's letter advised McDonald that he should be examined every two weeks and offered to transfer him anywhere in the continental United States. The letter also said, "Basically, regardless of your decision as to where you would like to go, you will be discharged on October 8, 1983." McDonald died 16 days after being flown to San Francisco. Silverman called the entire incident "a little bit baffling and a little bit tragic" (Odyssey, 1983).

Having to care for a patient with AIDS can be a frightening prospect, but the reluctance to treat AIDS may sometimes have reflected prejudice rather than justifiable fear of a serious disease. Dr. James W. Curran of the U.S. Public Health Service's Centers for Disease Control (CDC) wrote recently (Curran, 1983), "The past year has also been characterized by unwarranted hysteria over AIDS. Particularly disturbing are stories, although they are infrequent, about inadequate care given to patients with AIDS and the use of the syndrome as an excuse to justify discrimination." Since the great majority of people with AIDS are already regarded with some suspicion because they are homosexuals, drug users, or Haitian immigrants, health professionals must make a special effort to disentangle feelings of personal discomfort or disapproval from the legitimate caution they should exercise to avoid contracting AIDS themselves.

For all the worry and fear, few cases have been confirmed of health workers contracting AIDS from treating AIDS patients (CDC, 1983). However, because of the disease's long incubation period, the paucity of confirmed cases does not absolutely assure that few will turn up. Health professionals have a duty to exercise great care in handling blood and sputum samples from AIDS patients and, in general, to follow appropriate guidelines for infection control.

The final judgment on doctors and nurses must be that their avowed obligation to care for the sick extends to AIDS patients, regardless of personal fears. The moral force of a professional commitment to patients' health and welfare means nothing if the commitment is applied only when safe and convenient. People with AIDS often need special medical and nursing attention and deserve the same quality of care given any other patient. Exaggerated fears of a probably minimal danger of contracting AIDS are no excuse for failing to live up to professional vows.

Professional responsibility not only forbids the denial of treatment to AIDS patients, but includes the duty to respect the confidentiality of information patients may disclose in the course of treatment. It is implicitly understood that physicians and nurses may and should share information about a patient for the purpose of aiding the patient's medical treatment. Ruled out, though, are gossip, careless chatter in elevators and hallways, and other violations of the patient's privacy that do not contribute to patient care.

One important exception to the usual practice of respecting confidentiality is a state requirement that the disease or condition be reported. In virtually all states, gunshot wounds, suspected child abuse, and some sexually transmitted diseases must be reported. AIDS is now a reportable disease in over 30 states.

## MORAL RESPONSIBILITIES OF RESEARCHERS

Our greatest need is for continued research on AIDS—its treatment, cause, and prevention. Money has been allocated to the study of AIDS, and scientists are naturally attracted to attack a new puzzle like AIDS. Yet there has been one surprising, but important, impediment to AIDS research. The need to gather very sensitive information from the subjects of research faces the barrier of reluctance by potential subjects to reveal personal details out of fear that they might be used against them. In short, doubts about the protection of the confidentiality of research records, and a consequent lack of subjects' cooperation, have hampered AIDS research. Particularly affected is research on the epidemiology of AIDS—how it spreads. Epidemiologists must often ask personal questions, e.g., about sexual practices, drug use, and travel history.

All research on human subjects poses dangers. The three greatest concerns are respect for the rights of individual subjects, protection against unjustifiable harm, and the honoring of privacy. We respect their rights by requiring the informed consent of prospective subjects in advance of planned research, and by not allowing research on unknowing, incompetent, or coerced individuals. We protect them against unjustifiable harm by having a group of disinterested persons—the local Institutional Review Board—judge whether the risks of research are excessive. We respect privacy by ensuring that information learned about specific individuals is kept in confidence. The special problem in AIDS research is a heightened need for confidentiality because some of the most needed information is precisely the most sensitive and potentially dangerous that people can reveal about themselves.

The primary risk factors for AIDS include homosexuality, intravenous-drug use, and Haitian origin. Homosexual acts are illegal in many states, illicit drug use is illegal, by definition, in all states, and Haitians, like other recent immigrants, fear adverse action by the U.S. Immigration and Naturalization Service. The three high-risk groups have reason to fear that they are jeopardizing themselves by cooperating with researchers and revealing their names, residences, and other information. The recent disclosure to a blood bank of information from CDC files confirmed, for the gay community in particular, the risks of cooperating with AIDS research. People have expressed fears that such information may also be given to the FBI, CIA, Justice Department, and military services to the detriment of those who provided the information.

Still, the need for research is apparent, and many researchers and government officials recognize the problems. Dr. Edward N. Brandt, Jr., Assistant Secretary of Health and Human Services, has said (Krieger, 1983) "In investigating this disease, we've needed to examine and understand gay lifestyles. We've had to probe. Every disease raises the problem of confidentiality. But this disease raises it much more."

Representatives of the gay community have been especially active in raising questions about the confidentiality of research data. In a printed statement (Collins et al., undated)—"Who Knows What About Us?"—6 men, identifying themselves with the gay community, point to demands such as that by the conservative columnist Patrick Buchanan that homosexuals be banned from jobs involving food, health care, and contact with children. They describe scenarios in which federal or state agencies, such as the FBI and Drug Enforcement Administration, might try to obtain information about persons with AIDS, and conclude that "we as a community can no longer trust that the good intentions of others will adequately safeguard the confidentiality of information volunteered in good faith for research."

Despite grave reservations about giving sensitive information to researchers, some representatives of the gay community acknowledge the importance of research. Jeffrey Levi of the National Gay Task Force summed it up well (Marwick, 1983): "We could not be more interested in the gathering of information about AIDS. But we also firmly believe that reporting mechanisms must guarantee confidentiality."

The conflict could not be more clear or more tragic. The groups most at risk for contracting AIDS, with the most to gain from research, are at the same time hesitant to cooperate. Their hesitation is understandable in the light of the casual attitude researchers have too often taken toward the confidentiality of their data. Another factor impinging on confidentiality is that, except in a very few special categories such as some research on drug addiction and on crime, most research data are not well protected by either state or federal law. For the most part, the confidentiality of research records in the United States relies on the integrity of the researcher, including a willingness to face possible imprisonment should a court rule that the records must be disclosed.

One possible path out of this ethical morass is technology. There are many ways to disguise the identities of individuals in research. Names can be coded, parts of names deleted, and elaborate schemes erected to make it virtually or completely impossible to identify the subjects of research. However, no technological solution will work for all cases, and even under the best of circumstances, coding subjects' names would add to the expense and effort of research.

The problem must be solved in a way that wins the trust and promotes the candor of subjects suspicious of researchers and research agencies. A solution of sorts has been offered by The Hastings Center, which has asssembled a group involved in the controversy over research on AIDS—AIDS patients, representatives from the gay and Haitian communities, researchers, public health officials, and experts in law and ethics. This group has created guidelines for protecting confidentiality in AIDS research that are acceptable to all of the involved communities (Bayer et al., 1984). One feature of the guidelines is a review board that would address unresolved and newly emerging issues. This board would include representatives from all constituencies participating in the Hastings project.

## MORAL RESPONSIBILITIES OF PEOPLE WITH AIDS

AIDS poses a particularly severe moral challenge to the group most at risk—homosexuals. While it is not yet certain how AIDS is transmitted, it appears that sexual contact plays the most significant role in the gay community. In at least one homosexual subculture, promiscuity is a prominent feature of the lifestyle. It does not take much imagination to see that the very promiscuity that bolsters their sense of identity and raison d'etre is also probably their greatest threat.

The relation between sexual promiscuity and AIDS is not yet proven but seems very likely. If the relation does exist, what ethical issues arise from it? The issues for participants in the gay subculture pose questions for both those who have no AIDS symptoms and those with AIDS or its precursors. For those who do not have AIDS, prudence alone would require that they reconsider whether the pleasures of promiscuity are worth the risk. But is there a moral issue beyond this commonsensical advice? An increasingly popular theme is the responsibility people have for maintaining their own health.

In *The Mirage of Health* (Dubos, 1959), Rene Dubos argues that the great advances in health in the past century have been due more to public health improvements, such as sanitation and safe water, than to technological medicine. Certainly, medicine must be given its due, but it is a delusion to think we can keep doing things that make us ill and rely on medicine to restore us to health. The contemporary analogy, in the United States, to the improvement of sanitation and water cited by Dubos is probably the preservation and improvement of health by means of sensible diet, regular exercise, avoiding stress, stopping smoking, and getting enough rest, which may be more beneficial than the most sophisticated medical technologies. Likewise, the most effective way to prevent the spread of AIDS is to avoid activities that place people at risk.

Does this mean that people have a *moral* obligation to arrange their lives to avoid risks to health? The question of personal responsibility for individual health is far from settled. At one extreme, surely we are not required to avoid everything that poses the slightest risk. If there is any moral issue here, it must take into account the extent of the risk and the severity of the possible impact on health. At the other extreme, blatant carelessness that is almost certain to severely damage health may amount to moral irresponsibility.

Where AIDS and sexual promiscuity are concerned, the health risk is not yet known with enough certainty (though the consequences are certainly terrible) to permit the judgment that people are taking *immoral* risks with their health. Nor is it clear what would follow from such a judgment. For example, we do not deny medical care to people who overeat, smoke, or drive without fastening their seatbelts. Happily, evidence of beneficial changes in sexual behavior is being observed in studies that show declining gonorrhea rates among male homosexuals (Judson, 1983) and less promiscuity (Golubjatnikov et al., 1983).

For those with AIDS or its precursors who might transmit the disease to others, the moral questions are more compelling. Most important is the question of their responsibility to protect others. Some in the gay community regard calls for more "responsible" sexual behavior as a threat to the community's existence and values (Rechy, 1983), while others argue that it is both prudent and ethical to show restraint in a time of crisis (Lieberson, 1983). Since members of the gay community are at greatest risk, the debate has a special poignancy.

Actually, the issue of responsibility to refrain from spreading a sexually transmitted disease is an old question. However, the relative lethality of AIDS casts the issue in a new light. Of all the moral problems raised by AIDS, the most prominent may be the concern about blood. Curiously, most people—neither gay, Haitian, nor needle-employing drug users—can be comforted by the knowledge that they are almost certainly without danger of contracting AIDS. People who receive blood donated by individuals with AIDS (and possibly by those with AIDS precursors) appear to run some small risk of getting the disease. Since over 3,200,000 patients receive transfusions each year, an enormous population is exposed. Of course, only those given blood or blood products contaminated with AIDS incur any such risk. The simple fact is that we do not know for certain whether AIDS is transmitted through blood or, if it is, what proportion of exposed people actually get AIDS. Also, we do not know how much blood now in the supply network is capable of causing AIDS, nor can we clearly identify a potential donor whose blood may be dangerous to recipients.

Although there are many unknowns, we know enough to be concerned about the possible spread of AIDS through blood. The first ethical issues this concern raises have to do with the behavior of donors. Blood is given for many reasons, laudable ones, such as a desire to contribute to the general welfare, and more mundane ones, such as the desire to make money. Regardless of the motive for wanting to give blood, people who have reason to think their blood may transmit AIDS should refrain from donating to avoid endangering others. This principle may seem self-evident in the case of people with a confirmed diagnosis of AIDS; it is less clear in the case of others who are in high-risk groups but have no obvious symptoms of AIDS. The evidence, only suggestive at present, indicates that donors need not have overt AIDS to transmit it in their blood. The absence of symptoms is no guarantee that blood is safe. Until a reliable and sensitive screening procedure is developed, conservative policy dictates that all people with risk factors—homosexuals, drug users, and Haitians—be asked to refrain from giving blood (Bove, 1984). The success of this policy depends almost entirely on the voluntary cooperation of people in high-risk groups.

A controversy has grown up around one proposed method for avoiding the AIDS-by-transfusion danger—directed donation. With directed donation, blood is given by donors selected by a future recipient to be used solely for that recipient. This has some appeal for recipients who can summon a supply of safe, appropriately matched donors. However, the major U.S. blood-collecting organizations oppose directed donation, in part because it would lead to a two-track blood supply and discriminate against those who cannot locate willing donors, but also because even preselection of donors does not guarantee safety and because it increases the administrative burden. The problem of directed donation is complex and likely to be debated for some time.

## MORAL RESPONSIBILITIES OF SOCIETY

Among the many debates inspired by AIDS, one of the most difficult to judge is between those who believe that society is not doing nearly enough to study and control AIDS and those who believe that society is doing too much.

The question has no simple answer because there is no simple way to judge the ethics of resource-allocating decisions, especially when health is at stake. One commentator suggested that we could save more lives for the same money by giving air conditioners to the elderly poor than by doing research on AIDS. Whatever the truth of that suggestion, the fact is that allocation decisions generally defy moral logic. We spend nearly 200 million dollars to build an artificial heart, but cut preventive medicine programs, which cost a tiny fraction of that per person, even though those programs largely benefit the neediest.

If nothing else, the controversy over public money and AIDS may alert us to the moral confusion surrounding the spending of health dollars. Lacking a simple guide to how much money should be spent on AIDS, we can venture a complex principle—all members of the human community deserve efforts to spare them from disease and early death. If that requires an intensive effort against AIDS, so be it. But we cannot stop there. The same logic applies to other health needs of other populations. People with AIDS are not the only relatively powerless group; what is done for them should also be done for the poor, the elderly, and the children.

## SUMMARY

At least four groups have special moral responsibilities with respect to AIDS. First, health professionals, particularly physicians and nurses, have the same obligation to treat AIDS patients and respect their right to confidentially as they have toward all other patients. The fear that health professionals will contract AIDS in the line of duty is probably highly exaggerated, but, even if not, the obligation would still exist. Second, scientists doing research on AIDS have an especially strong obligation to respect personal confidentiality. Failure to fulfill this obligation may both invalidate present research and make it more difficult for others to gain the confidence of subjects of future research. Third, people with AIDS or exposed to AIDS have a moral responsibility to take reasonable precautions to protect their own health and the health of others, which may mean modifying sexual behavior or refraining from donating blood. Fourth, society has the same obligation to people with AIDS as it has to others who need assistance in the maintenance of health and treatment of illness.

# Four    Treating AIDS

# 12       Immune System Modulation in AIDS Therapy

## LEONARD SCARPINATO AND LEONARD CALABRESE

As described in an earlier chapter, the body's immune system can be viewed as an integrated network consisting of cell-mediated immunity, humoral (or antibody-mediated) immunity, complement, and phagocytes. The underlying immune defect of the acquired immune deficiency syndrome (AIDS) appears to be complex and multifactorial. Virtually all components of the body's immune system are affected, but cell-mediated immunity appears to be the most profoundly deranged. Cell-mediated immunity provides primary protection from viral, parasitic, and other opportunistic infections, as well as a surveillance system against the development of cancer. According to current understanding of the immune system, it also includes complex intercommunication among its various components through feedback mechanisms. These control mechanisms, which turn the immune response on and off, are severely disabled in AIDS. One need not understand the intricacies of the control mechanisms, but an appreciation of their existence is critical for understanding the problems facing medical scientists in developing treatments aimed at restoring a weakened immune system.

The most dramatic aspects of AIDS are the complicating infections and malignancies that actually cause the characteristic suffering and loss of life. While these complications characterize the disorder, it must be remembered that the most deadly feature of AIDS is also the most silent: the suppressed immune system. As its name implies, the disease is primarily a deficiency of the body's immunologic defenses. Infections and malignancies are the consequences of defective immunity. During phases of the illness when no infections or malignancies are apparent, individuals with AIDS may feel normal despite the underlying defective immunity. Many of the acute and life-threatening complications of AIDS can be successfully treated, but, unfortunately, the infections usually recur repeatedly until the patient ultimately succumbs. Clearly, successful treatment must be more than symptomatic; it must be directed at the root cause. Since it now appears that the human T-cell leukemia virus, HTLV-III, is responsible in whole or in part for AIDS, research is proceeding in two directions to combat it: first, development of specific antiviral therapies, including a preventive vaccine and effective therapeutic drugs; second, development of methods for reviving the ailing immune system.

## MODULATION OF CELL-MEDIATED IMMUNITY

Cellular immunity is mediated by the thymus-derived lymphocytes called T cells. These cells exert their effect in a complex fashion, critically dependent upon the secretion of and response to a number of hormonal products called lymphokines, which are secreted by lymphocytes. Two key lymphokines of current interest in AIDS are interleukin 2 (IL-2) and interferon.

T cells should be viewed as specialized bodies that attack invaders such as viruses, fungi, and parasites after they have entered host tissues. In AIDS, T cells cannot function properly, so infecting organisms may invade and persist in affected patients. Because IL-2 and interferon can boost T-cell and other types of immune functions (especially of natural killer cells), they are of great interest as potential therapeutic agents.

Before a therapeutic agent is accepted for human trial, several preliminary steps must be completed. First experimental evidence, either in the test tube or in animals, must indicate that the agent may successfully combat the disease in question. Second, evidence must be acquired, usually by animal experiments, to indicate that the drug or modality is safe for human use. After these criteria are met, the treatment is ready for what is known as a Phase I trial, which attempts to establish safety and the appropriate dose for human patients. Only after these steps are completed can the drug be subjected to therapeutic trials of effectiveness. It is no wonder then, in light of these requirements and the relatively recent arrival of AIDS, that successful experimental trials and therapies have been slow in coming.

**Interleukin 2**

IL-2, which is deficient in AIDS patients, is capable of restoring lymphocytic ability to kill virus-infected cells. This is particularly relevant since most investigators feel that AIDS is probably due to a viral agent. Furthermore, since IL-2 is a natural product of the body, it appears to be relatively safe in early studies. IL-2 is now undergoing Phase I trials in several centers, but results are not yet conclusive. One major drawback in the trial of IL-2 is its current availability in only minute amounts, which hampers its study on a wide scale.

**Interferon**

Interferon has performed exciting feats in the test tube and has been shown to modify the natural course of certain chronic viral infections in humans. Reports of Phase I trials of interferon in AIDS patients with Kaposi's sarcoma are encouraging. In one study of 12 patients, major tumor regression was noted in 5, partial regression in 3, and no significant response in 4. In another study, 14 of 35 patients showed marked tumor regression and also had a low incidence of opportunistic infections. Additionally, interferon was relatively free of side effects and improved several immunologic functions. Unlike IL-2, interferon is available in quantity for study and has been used with some success in other forms of cancer. However, it should be noted that an abnormal interferon is found in increased amounts in many patients with AIDS, prompting some observers to suggest that this interferon variant may be an immunosuppressive agent. Moreover, while early trials suggested that interferon was somewhat effective in the treatment of Kaposi's sarcoma, not all patients responded favorably, the results were not significantly better than with conventional chemotherapy, and some follow-up studies have failed to show even marginal benefits.

Some experts have advocated combining interferon and IL-2 in therapy. This has strong theoretical support and will no doubt be tried in the near future. Studies are now under way in AIDS-related-complex patients to see whether interferon and/or IL-2 can prevent the occurrence of overt AIDS.

### Bone Marrow Transplantation/Lymphocyte Transfusion

Bone marrow, located in the inner portion of bones, contains cells that develop into blood cells, and also contains the stem cells of T and B lymphocytes. Bone marrow transplantation (BMT) is the treatment for a variety of blood disorders, including aplastic anemia and certain leukemias. In BMT, performed under sterile conditions in an operating room, a needle is passed through a donor's skin into a hip bone in an area called the iliac crest. Bone marrow is aspirated (prevented from clotting with heparin, a blood thinner) and then infused into the recipient through a vein. The transplanted cells circulate in the bloodstream, settle in the recipient's bone marrow, and grow.

There are distinct immunologic markers, called HLA antigens, present on most cells of the body. These enable the body to distinguish its own from other cells so that foreign cells with incorrect HLA markers can be singled out for destruction. Normally, when unmatched HLA cells are infused, the recipient's immune system destroys the donor's stem cells; otherwise the donor's cells could attack the recipient's cells. Immunosuppressive drugs are given during BMT to prevent such a reaction. The only time this is unnecessary is with identical twins, since their HLA markers are also identical.

Thus, BMT could theoretically give an AIDS patient new stem cells to rebuild the immune system and alleviate the underlying immune defect. This has been tried at least once. In a set of identical twins, one of whom was a homosexual with AIDS, bone marrow was taken from the healthy heterosexual twin and given to his brother. The AIDS twin experienced some improvement in his helper/suppressor T-cell ratio and also developed a positive skin test response, which had been negative before the transfusion, thus indicating improvement in T-cell function. However, he was not cured and eventually succumbed to his disease. Dr. Clifford Lane and his group, who performed this experiment at the National Institute of Health

(NIH), is still hopeful that their results will be of value in designing further efforts to bolster the immune systems of AIDS patients.

By a procedure similar to BMT, the lymphocytes of a donor can be infused into an AIDS recipient, except that the cell source is not the marrow but the circulating blood in the veins. When tried in one AIDS patient, it resulted only in a short-lived lymphocytosis (increase in the number of lymphocytic white blood cells) with no change in the patient's clinical conditions. BMT is often accompanied by a lymphocyte transfusion in an attempt to increase the chance of success.

Obviously, BMT experimentation is not complete, but there is hope that, after further trials and research, this form of therapy may help AIDS patients in the future.

### Transfer Factor

Transfer factor (TF) is basically an extract of lymphocytes from one or more donors that is capable of transferring skin test reactivity from an immunocompetent donor to an immunologically naive recipient. TF has been used with limited success in certain immunodeficiency diseases such as chronic mucocutaneous candidiasis. Investigators in Cleveland, Ohio, at Case Western Reserve University and the Cleveland Clinic, are now making TF from clinically stable patients with HTLV-III infection and giving it to patients with AIDS. The results of these experiments are too preliminary to comment on.

## MECHANICAL THERAPY

### Plasmapheresis

The suffix in the term plasmapheresis is derived from the Greek word meaning "to take away." In practice, plasmapheresis is the removal of the fluid elements of the blood (plasma) followed by return of the blood cells to the patient. This type of therapy is potentially useful when certain disease-causing substances travel in the circulation. It is relatively safe and has proved to be beneficial for a variety of disorders. In AIDS, several abnormal elements have been found in the blood, including potentially harmful agents such as immune complexes and acid-labile interferon. Dr. Jeffry Laurence and colleagues have identified a soluble immunosuppressive substance in the plasma of most AIDS patients that may contribute to the underlying immune defect. On the basis of these findings and the lack of specific knowledge of the factors related to the cause of AIDS, the empiric application of plasma exchange has been attempted on a number of patients with transient lymphocyte increase but no disease cure.

## MODULATING THYMUS FUNCTION

The thymus is the most essential gland for converting lymphocytes, produced in the bone marrow, into T cells. Located in the chest near the heart, the thymus is sometimes so large in children that it causes concern of a possible tumor, but shrinks and blends so well with other tissues in adults that it is sometimes difficult to find during surgery. Accordingly, the functional importance of this gland was thought to diminish with age.

However, research over the last 10 years has discovered that hormone-like chemicals are released by the thymus throughout life. These chemicals were first found in a rough extract, or "parent compound," made of ground-up thymus glands from calves. Initially studied in laboratory animals and in the test tube, this extract was eventually used successfully on humans—children at first—with special immunologic defects somewhat like those seen in AIDS. Over the years, the parent compound has been found by laborious purification techniques to contain many different substances. These substances are: thymopoietin II (TP), facteur thymique serique (FTS, thymulin), thymic humoral factor (THF), thymic Factor X (TFX), thymosin alpha 1, thymosin fraction 5, thymopentin (TPS), and suppressin. Although all enhance the immune system in some fashion, the two affected by AIDS are thymosin alpha 1 and thymulin (FTS).

### Thymosin Alpha 1

Scientists know the chemical structure of thymosin alpha 1 and can measure blood levels by radioimmunoassay. Recent studies have shown elevated levels in AIDS patients, levels that may not be effective, so the patients were given purified thymosin fraction 5. Unfortunately, although it restored the response to some tests of immunity, it did not help to alleviate the disease. At George Washington University, Dr. Goldstein and his colleagues have now given thymosin fraction 5 to people with AIDS-related complex and are watching to see if it prevents them from progressing to AIDS.

### Thymulin

FTS concentrations in the blood of AIDS patients were found to be subnormal. This was discovered in France and is now under investigation.

### Thymus Transplantation

Another approach has been thymus transplantation. A part of the thymus gland is first taken from a young child, usually during heart surgery when the chest is open. Then, after complicated preparation, the thymus tissue is transplanted under the skin of the recipient, usually in the forearm. It takes several weeks to evaluate a graft. Thymus transplantation has been used with moderate success for a number of childhood or genetic immunodeficiencies. Clinicians at Yale University led by Dr. John Dwyer have now performed at least 16 thymus transplants on AIDS patients. As of November 1984, there was enough evidence to show this treatment alone will not cure AIDS. A significant but transient rise in T-cell function occurred but all eventually succumbed to infection which dropped the T cell numbers. Currently transplants with subsequent IL-2 infusions are being attempted.

### OTHER MODALITIES

### Cytomegalovirus Vaccine

At present, several viruses have been found to be universally present in AIDS patients and are suspected of at least contributing to the underlying immune defect. A successful vaccine against any or all of these agents may prove beneficial. Accordingly, the development of a cytomegalovirus (CMV) vaccine now has a high priority.

Work has been done on the CMV vaccine at various centers since around 1973. The vaccine showing the most promise is called Towne-125. Trials have taken place, and the Federal Drug Administration is now trying to decide whether this vaccine will be beneficial and, if so, for how long. At present, the vaccine is not available to physicians. Given the difficulties already encountered in vaccine development and the previous experience with hepatitis B and polio, it may be 5–10 years before a successful vaccine is ready for use.

### Acyclovir

It is obviously highly desirable to have not only a preventive CMV vaccine but also an antiviral agent that could kill CMV after an infection has started. It initially appeared that an antiherpes agent called acyclovir (Zovirax) might be useful against CMV and the Epstein-Barr virus (another virus often found in AIDS patients). It is now evident that the dosage required to produce an appreciable effect approaches a toxic level.

### Recent Drug Therapies

In recent years, many drugs have been found to have a beneficial effect on the immune system and are thus potentially useful for treating AIDS. Unfortunately, they have tended to be immunopotentiating in the test tube, but fall short when used against actual immunodeficiency disease. For example, cimetidine, a drug used to treat peptic ulcers, restores a positive skin-test response in certain people who have Candida infections but do not respond to Candida skin tests. However, the drug seems to have no curative action against infections caused by the fungus.

The following are some drugs that have shown promise in the laboratory but have not yet proved to be effective against clinical immunodeficiency (although they may be useful in the treatment of other conditions): cimetidine, isoprinosine, procainamide, azimexion (experimental), histamine, and indomethacin. Several of these drugs have been shown to enhance the action of other immunomodulators. Another drug, tunicamycin, increases the antiviral and anticellular effect of interferon.

### NUTRITION AND THE IMMUNE SYSTEM

Adequate nutrition is essential for good health and normal body function, including that of the immune system. Although there is no evidence that good nutrition can enhance immune responsiveness, there is much evidence that poor nutrition can decrease it. In a well-balanced diet, the nutrients discussed below are present in sufficient quantities for proper functioning of the immune system.

Among the nutrients whose lack can adversely affect the immune response are vitamins A and C, certain lipids and amino acids, glucose, and zinc. For example, there is good evidence, both laboratory and clinical, that zinc is important for cell-mediated immunity. An inadequate zinc intake and consequent low level of blood zinc are associated with a decrease in both T-cell abundance and function. Zinc therapy restores the immune response in patients with zinc-related immunodeficiencies. Although zinc levels have not been studied in AIDS patients, the need for an adequate dietary intake of zinc (or a multivitamin supplement for a poor diet) is indicated. Laboratory evidenc˙ also suggests that vitamin C enhances interferon production.

High-risk individuals should be especially prudent about eating sufficient (but not excessive) amounts of essential nutrients. Patients hospitalized with AIDS or AIDS-related complex are sometimes found to be malnourished. The physician may then give nutrients intravenously either through a small peripheral vein in a hand or arm, or through a larger vein in the groin or neck. Such intravenous feeding, called hyperalimentation or total parenteral nutrition, can save patients' lives by safely fulfilling the nutritional needs of the body and its immune system.

## UNPROVEN AND UNCONVENTIONAL THERAPIES

### Megadose Vitamins

There is no proof that massive doses of vitamins can affect or cure AIDS. Certain vitamins are required, but not in mega (very large) doses. Not only is their efficacy unproven, but megadoses of vitamins may be deleterious because of harmful side effects.

### Laetrile

An extract from apricot pits, Laetrile was originally touted as a cure for cancer. Although it failed in clinical studies and is not approved for use in the United States, it is still available, usually at high cost, in some foreign countries. Laetrile has resurfaced as a possible therapy for AIDS, but there is neither proof of its effectiveness against AIDS or AIDS-associated opportunistic infections and malignancies nor any theoretical basis for its use.

### Reticuloendothelial Vaccine

Advertisements in gay-oriented newspapers imply that reticuloendothelial vaccine (REV) can prevent AIDS. The vaccine is advertised as very "scientific," with the claim that rabbits are used to form antibodies that stimulate and normalize the reticuloendothelial system, the part of the immune system that engulfs and destroys antigens. This vaccine can be dangerous because the rabbit material may trigger an anaphylactic response (an exaggerated body reaction to foreign substances, that restricts the flow of air and blood) or serum sickness (an allergic blood reaction). REV, which is available only in some foreign countries, is backed by no scientific proof of benefits in the prevention or cure of AIDS.

### Stress Reduction, Acupuncture, and Oriental Herbs

Although not generally harmful, stress reduction, acupuncture, and oriental herbs have not been shown to cure AIDS. They and other therapies may sometimes give subjective relief—the patient feels better but is not cured or freed of symptoms.

These treatments become harmful only when used to exclude medical treatment. If specific medical treatments for some AIDS infections are delayed or ignored, the outcome may be fatal.

In the Alternative Therapy Unit at San Francisco General Hospital (probably the only such unit in the United States), the focus is on making AIDS patients feel as comfortable as possible. Although no claims are made about improving immune responses, Dr. Dorothy Waddell (physician), Ms. Deirdre Claiborn (acupuncturist), and Ms. Jean Sayre-Adams (nurse) state that AIDS patients tolerate the disease and treatment better in this environment. The unit's directors use a variety of therapies, including oriental herbs (Chinese medicine), acupuncture, Simonton's therapeutic touch, counseling, meditation, and visualizations. They report that these therapies are always given as adjuncts to medical treatment.

### Anti-HTLV-III Therapy

With the discovery that human T-cell leukemia virus (HTLV-III) is the likely cause of AIDS (in whole or in part), new therapeutic efforts have been mounted directly against the presumed etiologic agent. The greatest hope lies in the development of a vaccine that would induce lasting immunity and thus prevent the disease. Although vaccine development is proceeding, it faces major obstacles, including the facts that no vaccine has ever successfully been produced against a retrovirus, and that AIDS infections are complex and may not be warded off by a specific antibody.

Another goal of development is an antiviral drug to help those already infected. Suramin, which has inhibited HTLV-III infectivity and replication in the test tube, is now being tested in AIDS patients.

## SUMMARY

There is not yet any proven therapy for AIDS that corrects the underlying immune deficit, but many avenues of research are being explored. At present, the primary treatment medical science has to offer is directed at the complications of immunocompromise, namely antimicrobials for the infections and conventional chemotherapy, and some attempts at immunotherapy, for the malignancies.

Attempts at immunomodulation in the treatment of AIDS include the use of interleuken 2, interferon, bone marrow transplants, plasmapharesis, thymus extracts and transplantation, CMV vaccine, acyclovir, drugs affecting T cells, improved nutrition, and various unproven and unconventional therapies.

# Five

Avoiding or Coping with AIDS

# 13       Caring for the AIDS Patient
## MARY E. CUFF

The health-care needs of individuals with acquired immune deficiency syndrome (AIDS) change during the course of the illness and must often be met in a variety of settings. The care providers also vary and may be the individual himself, professional nurses, home health aides, family, or friends.

Typically, the AIDS patient experiences multiple hospitalizations for treatment of acute opportunistic infections. In the hospital, of course, the primary care provider is a professional nurse. Between acute episodes, the patient may be able to resume normal activities and take responsibility for self-care. In later, debilitating or terminal stages of the disease, family and friends may elect to provide care at home with the help of visiting nurses or home health aides. AIDS presents especially difficult problems for the patient and attendants, as indicated in table 1.

Care of the AIDS patient depends on types and severity of infections and malignancies that accompany the disease, and on the extent of physical debilitation brought on by chronic diarrhea, malnutrition, fevers, and complications of therapy. The patient is also likely to have profound emotional needs, not only because of an awareness that the disease may be fatal and possibly transmitted to friends and family, but also because victims come largely from socially stigmatized groups. Individual emotional responses to AIDS of course vary with inherent coping abilities, spiritual strengths and beliefs, the availability of support from family, friends, and others, and the degree of illness.

## TABLE 1.   CARE PROBLEMS FREQUENTLY ENCOUNTERED WITH AIDS PATIENTS

| Problem | Related Factors |
| --- | --- |
| Respiratory distress<br>Inability to supply oxygen to<br>   tissues | *Pneumocystis carinii* pneumonia<br>Respiratory and other opportunistic<br>   infections<br>Anxiety |
| Malnutrition<br>Dehydration | Chronic diarrhea<br>Lesions of the mouth and esophagus<br>Kaposi's sarcoma of the gastro<br>   intestinal tract<br>Nausea and vomiting induced by<br>   medications<br>Increased metabolic rate with fevers<br>Depression of chronic illness |
| Mental changes<br>Sensory or motor impairment<br>Potential for accidental injury | Social and physical isolation<br>Psychological response to catastrophic<br>   illness<br>Infections or malignancies of the<br>   central nervous system |
| Social isolation<br>Loss of control/powerlessness<br>Disturbance in self-perception<br>Anxiety/fear | Imposed isolation requirements<br>Community/family/health-care<br>   personnel's attitudes<br>Physical dependency<br>Poor prognosis<br>Symptoms of acute infections |
| Inability to provide proper home<br>   care | Lack of community support services<br>Inadequate home-care information<br>Lack of people to assist with care |

The following discussion of the needs of the AIDS patient is divided into acute care in the hospital and home care, with references to chronic problems that require attention throughout the course of the disease.

## HOSPITAL CARE

AIDS patients are usually admitted to a hospital for treatment of life-threatening opportunistic infections. These infections are caused by organisms, common in the environment, that have little effect on a healthy person with normal immune defenses, but may produce severe illness when the immune system is deficient, as in AIDS. On admission to the hospital, AIDS patients are often acutely ill, physically debilitated, and apprehensive.

### Objectives

The objectives of care for the hospitalized AIDS patient are:

Identification and treatment of infections
Maintaining the function of affected organs
Symptomatic relief
Prevention or early detection of complications related to treatment
Improvement of general well-being
Compassionate mental and emotional support

The first step is an assessment of the patient's physical and emotional condition (see table 2), which includes interviews with appropriate health-care professionals, a physical examination, and various diagnostic procedures and laboratory tests. These may be disturbing to patients who are physically and emotionally exhausted by their illness. Health-care personnel should explain the necessity for the assessment and be especially sensitive to concerns about the confidentiality of divulged information. Assurances should be given that such information will be kept private and shared only when necessary to benefit the patient's treatment.

Care is then planned on the basis of the assessment. The plan focuses first on the most critical problems, which, in most cases, are opportunistic infections and malfunction of infected organs.

**TABLE 2.   ADMISSION ASSESSMENT OF THE AIDS PATIENT**

Patient's description of the nature, onset, and duration of acute symptoms prior to hospitalization, including:
   Respiratory distress, shortness of breath, rapid breathing, or nonproductive cough
   Headache, neck stiffness, or sensitivity to light accompanied by nausea and vomiting
   Changes in thought processes or behavior noted by family or friends
   Changes in vision, hearing, balance, or mobility
   Loss of appetite, volume and frequency of diarrhea, nausea, vomiting, and extent of weight loss
   Fevers or night sweats
   Lesions on skin or in the mouth
   Ability to perform normal daily activities

A review of patient's medical history and related events, including:
   Occurrence and onset of prodromal symptoms such as lymph-node enlargement, fevers, night sweats, viral-like illnesses
   History of sexually transmitted diseases, parasitic and other types of infection requiring treatment
   Recent blood transfusions
   Recent travel, especially outside the country

A discussion of psychosocial factors that influence the illness or hospitalization, including:
   Sexual preference
   Recreational drug use
   Response to acute illness, including expectations of hospitalization and degree of anxiety and expressed fears
   Availability of emotional support from family or others
   Availability of financial and social support

A physical examination to establish baseline function of major organ systems, with particular attention to systems subject to infection, including:
   Neurological—evaluation of thought processes and sensory or motor defects
   Respiratory—ability of the lungs to exchange oxygen
   Skin—lesions related to infection or malignancy
   Gastrointestinal—motility of the intestines and the presence of malignant growths

**TABLE 2.    (continued)**

Diagnostic and laboratory tests, including:
  Complete blood count, including the numbers and types of white blood
    cells
  Blood chemistry
  Blood gas analysis—oxygen-carbon dioxide balance
  Antibody titers—signs of recent exposure to infections
  Chest and abdominal x-rays

Also included may be:
  Bronchoscopy—to examine lung tissue for infection or malignancy
  Spinal tap—to examine spinal fluid for CNS infections
  Endoscopy—to directly examine the gastrointestinal tract
  CAT scans of the brain—to detect lesions or infection


**Lung Infection**

The most common opportunistic infection of AIDS, requiring hospitalization and skilled nursing care, is *Pneumocystis carinii* pneumonia (PCP). Usually symptoms include rapid, labored breathing, a
nonproductive cough, and extreme anxiety because of an inability to
draw enough oxygen from the air into the bloodstream. Immediate
care consists of relieving respiratory distress, supplementing the oxygen supply to the tissues, and drug therapy to inhibit continued
growth of the infecting organism.

Symptoms may be relieved by the administration of high concentrations of oxygen through a face mask. However, some patients
with advanced pneumonia may need more intensive support from a
respirator machine connected to an endotracheal tube placed in the
windpipe. The respirator delivers high concentrations of oxygen directly to the lung and reduces the effort required to breathe. Since the
procedure can be frightening to an already anxious patient and also
causes some physical discomfort, the care provider should give reassuring explanations of its necessity and benefits. It is also important
to explain that the tube prevents speaking, and to provide a pad the
patient can write on.

Drug therapy for PCP is usually a combination of trimethoprim
and sulfamethoxazole (TMP-SMX), administered intravenously, or

pentamidine, an experimental drug available only from the Centers for Disease Control. While remissions of PCP may occur, these drugs are not without significant side effects that might require their discontinuation. TMP-SMX may cause kidney problems, nausea, vomiting, severe rashes, and sometimes an impaired ability to produce certain blood cells, such as platelets, necessary for blood clotting, and granulocytes, white blood cells that fight bacterial infections. Pentamidine may impair kidney and liver function, decrease the production of white blood cells, and produce painful abcesses at injection sites. Intravenous infusion of pentamidine may cause a sudden drop in blood pressure and a rapid pulse rate. Drug therapy must be accompanied by close monitoring, including blood tests, pressure measurements, and careful personal observation.

Acute respiratory distress often provokes severe anxiety and fear of dying. Also, the isolation by some hospitals of AIDS patients on respirators intensifies feelings of social ostracism. Relaxation exercises and controlled breathing techniques often help to alleviate some symptoms. Exploring fears with the patient may help to reduce them. Sometimes the most effective therapy is the simplest—the concern and comforting presence of a caring person, which is at least as important as technical monitoring. If the hospital does require patient isolation, the care provider should make sure that all concerned understand the basis for such a precaution.

*P. carinii* is regarded by most authorities as an inactive parasite present in the lung tissue of more than 90% of adults. Only when the immune system is severely compromised is this organism able to multiply and produce a life-threatening lung infection. Pneumonia caused by this organism is virtually nonexistent among healthy adults, and health-care workers and healthy visitors are not at risk of contracting it from a PCP patient. However, in acute-care settings many patients have suppressed immunity for various reasons. It is remotely possible that those caring for a patient with PCP could inhale droplets containing the organism and transmit it to other patients with immune deficiencies. While such transmission is considered unlikely, health-care providers may wear face masks as an added precaution. Visitors who are unlikely to make contact with immunosuppressed patients elsewhere in the hospital usually do not have to wear masks.

Additional measures to deal with potential social isolation will be discussed below.

### Central Nervous System Infection

The central nervous system (CNS) is the second most common site of acute infections in AIDS patients. The most frequent are cryptococcosis (due to a fungus from weathered pigeon droppings) and toxoplasmosis (due to a parasite excreted by cats). Meningitis (inflammation of membranes of the brain and spinal cord) and encephalitis (inflamation of the brain itself) may be caused by a number of different organisms. Less common are primary CNS lymphoma and a viral syndrome called progressive multifocal leukoencephalopathy (PML).

The signs and symptoms of CNS infections are especially distressing to the patient and family. They often include severe headaches, sensitivity to light, neck stiffness, vomiting, fevers, and sometimes seizures and loss of some sensory or motor functions. A loss of vision or the ability to maintain balance increases the dependence of patients on care providers and is a frustrating reminder of their disease. Discomfort may be alleviated by a dark, quiet environment and medication to control vomiting and fevers. Medications to control seizures often make the patient drowsy and distort perception. Seizures or motor defects require precautions to assure patient safety, e.g., padded siderails, urging the patient to call for help in walking, and keeping the surroundings free of clutter. However, patients may also find these precautions restrictive.

Occasionally, CNS infections or malignancies cause changes in behavior and mental confusion that are very disturbing to the family and friends of young, previously normal individuals. These dismayed witnesses may need professional assurance that alterations in the patient's personality are uncontrollable consequences of the infection.

Changes in behavior and mental ability may be so great that the AIDS patient can no longer maintain personal hygiene or react properly to prevent injury. This may necessitate 24-hour attendance for an extended period, which can drastically increase the financial burden of treatment. Also, the need for others to maintain the patient's personal hygiene intensifies his feelings of helplessness and dependency. The professionals who must tend to a disabled patient's hygiene can help to lessen these feelings by making sure to give help in private and by encouraging the patient to be as self-sufficient as possible. The exercise by the patient of some control over these tasks can go far to diminish the sense of total powerlessness.

The loss of bowel and bladder control with advanced CNS disease increases the risk of contamination of linens and equipment with body fluids. This requires extra isolation precautions, including the wearing of gowns and gloves by personnel when in the patient's room. It is important to emphasize here that isolation procedures are intended to reduce the risk of exposure to blood or body fluids that may harbor AIDS virus. CNS infections are not themselves transmitted by person-to-person contact and do not require patient isolation when not associated with AIDS.

Medical treatment for the CNS infection includes potent drugs with potentially toxic effects. Amphoteracin B, used to treat fungal infections such as cryptococcal meningitis, may cause fever and chills, a decrease in blood pressure, an increase in heart rate, chest pain, muscle weakness, and impaired kidney function. Medication for treating toxoplasmosis may decrease the ability of the bone marrow to produce adequate numbers of blood cells, among other possible side effects.

### Malnutrition and Dehydration

Malnutrition and dehydration are recurrent problems for the AIDS patient, both in the hospital and at home. One of the most troublesome causes is chronic, persistent diarrhea, which may be due to viral or parasitic infections, malignancies involving the gastrointestinal tract, or unidentified causes. Massive diarrhea, up to 17 liters a day, sometimes occurs with Cryptosporidium infections.

Exacerbating the nutritional problems of AIDS patients are loss of appetite, nausea, and vomiting due to treatment with antibiotics or chemotherapy. Lesions in the mouth and esophagus from Kaposi's sarcoma or Candida or herpes infections often make swallowing painful and decrease the desire for food. At the same time, fevers may significantly increase the metabolic rate and increase caloric requirements.

The factors that combine to produce malnutrition often result in extreme weight loss, wasting of muscle tissue, and loss of skin tone. Tissue healing and repair are adversely affected by an inadequate protein intake. Malnutrition also impairs the immune system, further suppressing the AIDS patient's ability to withstand infection.

The objectives of care for the malnourished patient are:

Identification of the source of diarrhea or malabsorption, and appropriate treatment
Alleviation of distressing symptoms
An increase in protein and calorie intake
Restoration of fluid balance
A decrease in metabolic caloric demands

Medical treatment for the underlying cause of malnutrition is not always available or effective. Many responsible organisms are difficult to identify. Others, such as Cryptosporidium, were rarely seen in man prior to the AIDS epidemic, and effective drug therapy has not yet been developed. Treatment, therefore, is frequently limited to symptomatic relief.

Some drugs, such as Kaopectate, that act locally in the intestine to absorb toxic substances and protect the intestinal wall, may be partially effective in controlling chronic diarrhea. More frequently used for the diarrhea of AIDS are systemic drugs, containing narcotics, that slow the movement of food through the intestinal tract and increase the tone of the intestinal wall. However, they often achieve only temporary improvement.

Antiemetics, used to decrease nausea and vomiting, may be helpful when administered before meals or before the giving of medication known to induce vomiting. The control of nausea and a change to small frequent feedings usually increase food consumption and the absorption of nutrients. Local anesthetic gels applied to mouth sores, and the avoidance of hot, cold, or spicy foods can ease the pain of swallowing, improve appetite, and increase food intake.

If malnutrition is not too severe, the patient may be able to gain weight with high calorie-high protein drinks recommended by a nutritionist. However, these high calorie drinks contain concentrated glucose which, in some patients, promotes water absorption into the intestine and consequent watery stools or diarrhea.

More severe malnutrition, especially in patients who are unable to swallow, requires liquid feeding through a tube inserted through the nose and into the stomach. Such liquid feedings may also induce diarrhea, particularly if large volumes of a concentrated glucose-protein solution are administered too quickly. Diluting the solution and feeding by slow and continuous infusion usually eliminate this problem.

Patients unable to absorb nutrients through the gastrointestinal tract may be given concentrated glucose-protein solutions intravenously (hyperalimentation). Intake directly into the bloodstream may exceed 5,000 calories per day and usually produces rapid improvement. Since hyperalimentation requires the insertion of a catheter into a major blood vessel, the major risk is infection, always a special threat to AIDS patients. Not only is the skin penetrated, but highly concentrated glucose solutions are an excellent medium for the growth of bacteria, which then have direct access to the bloodstream through the intravenous catheter. Extreme care must be taken by health-care personnel to prevent infection as well as to monitor the patient's nutritional condition.

A malnourished patient must also be helped to expend less energy to decrease caloric requirements and conserve nutrients for vital functions. For example, a fever increases the metabolic rate approximately 7% for each degree above normal temperature, and a prolonged fever can significantly deplete available energy. A feverish patient is given acetaminophen (Tylenol) and temperature is closely monitored as part of nutritional management. If fevers resist control with acetaminophen, or are extremely high, a cooling blanket may be applied to lower body temperature. The rapid breathing and heart rate that accompany fevers, drug reactions, and anxiety also consume calories. Teaching the patient relaxation techniques and controlled breathing exercises is a beneficial adjunct to medical treatment.

### Isolation Precautions—Effect on Patient Morale

The AIDS patient has special problems that arise from isolation requirements for a potentially transmissible disease. Both care providers and patients should thoroughly appreciate the reasons for precautions to avoid unnecessary misunderstandings.

Available evidence suggests that AIDS is caused by a virus transmitted through sexual contact or blood products. Although their risk appears to be very small, it is reasonable that care providers take precautions against exposure to AIDS patients' blood and body fluids. AIDS patients admitted to a hospital are placed in a category of isolation known as "Blood and Body Fluid Precautions." These precautions, recommended by the Centers for Disease Control, are discussed in detail in Chapter 14.

Secondary infections or complications sometimes require modification of the basic precautions. While the majority of secondary infections seen with AIDS are not transmissible to a healthy individual, other patients in a hospital may have impaired immunity and be more susceptible. Health-care workers are in frequent contact with many of these patients and must take extra precautions against conveying an infection from one patient to another. One example of extra precautions, mentioned earlier, is respiratory isolation and the wearing of face masks for PCP. Face masks are also worn for patients with tuberculosis or other potentially transmissible respiratory infections. It should be emphasized again that it is not necessary to wear masks while caring for an AIDS patient if transmissible respiratory infections are absent. There is no evidence at all that AIDS virus can be transmitted through the air.

Immunosuppressed patients, including those with AIDS, are especially vulnerable to herpesvirus infections, which may cause painful lesions over large areas of the skin. The fluid in these lesions is highly infectious and often contaminates linen and nearby surfaces. Isolation precautions are more stringent, if patients have such extensive infections, to prevent care providers from inadvertently transmitting infectious material to other immunosuppressed patients. Both visitors and health-care workers may develop herpes infections if they come into contact with the fluids from herpes lesions, although such infections will be much less severe. Additional isolation precutions include wearing gowns and gloves at all times, use of a private room, and covering lesions with a moistureproof dressing whenever the patient must leave the room.

Further precautions are necessary if the patient loses bowel or bladder control, or is mentally incapable of complying with cautionary advice. Such precautions were described above in relation to CNS infections.

Modifications discussed thus far have additions to basic precautions. If the AIDS patient has no transmissible secondary infections, precautions may be relaxed. Care providers may enter the patient's room without putting on special gowns or gloves if they do not have to handle blood or be exposed to body fluids. Also AIDS patients capable of self-care and free of transmissible infection may share a room with other patients as long as separate bathroom facilities are available.

While care providers must be concerned with appropriate isolation precautions to avoid exposure to the AIDS virus and to prevent transmission of secondary infections to other patients, they should have equal concern to protect the AIDS patient against the adverse effects of isolation. Feelings of being an outcast, loss of control, and diminished self-esteem, frequent in most AIDS patients, are heightened by isolation imposed during hospitalization. Patients may also be depressed if family and friends withdraw because they dread the diagnosis, cannot cope with a debilitating disease, and fear the eventual loss of a loved one. A patient may also create isolation by choosing not to discuss the illness or problems of lifestyle with family, friends, and co-workers.

Unconscious avoidance of health-care personnel and decreased opportunities for casual contact may result from the time-consuming demands of isolation procedures. Care providers, too, may distance themselves to avoid the pain of losing a patient they have become close to. Finally, despite extensive programs to educate health-care workers about the realities of AIDS transmission, a few still avoid AIDS patients for fear of contracting the disease or because of prejudice against members of the high-risk groups.

### Psychosocial Support

The responsibility of the professional nurse is to provide a setting with social and environmental stimulation, to help the patient find inner resources and external sources of support, and to educate family, friends, and other health-care workers regarding appropriate isolation practices.

Helping the patient to interact positively with others can include a conscious effort to visit often, even when there are no specific tasks to perform, spending more time with the patient, and not only talking but touching and otherwise communicating acceptance and personal concern. Ambulatory patients who do not require isolation should be encouraged to leave their rooms and use common patient areas. When the patient must be confined to the room, radio, television, and reading materials may increase the feeling of contact with the outside world and provide distraction from immediate concerns.

Support groups for people with AIDS have been established in many metropolitan areas in the United States (see Chapter 17 for a list of local referral centers). Patients who do not wish to avail themselves of such support groups should be urged to seek individual counseling or spiritual support to help cope with their disease. (Chapter 15 gives a detailed discussion of support systems and strategies.)

The professional health-care provider must assume the role of educator to promote optimum care for AIDS patients. Fear of AIDS will continue to plague its victims until it is established without question that AIDS is not highly transmissible and does not pose a threat to the general population. Professional care providers must not only convey the known facts about AIDS to patients, families, other health-care workers, and the public, but must also confront and correct misinformation to change inappropriate responses to AIDS patients.

## HOME CARE

Care may be provided in the home during three phases of AIDS: when the patient is free of serious infection and able to perform normal daily activities; when the patient is debilitated by chronic illness and requires considerable assistance; and the terminal phase of the disease.

### Objectives

The objectives of home care vary somewhat with the phase of the disease, but the following are likely to apply at one time or another:

Avoid patient exposure to infectious environmental organisms
Alleviate concerns of patient and those close to the patient regarding transmission of infection or AIDS
Maintain or improve nutritional state

Obtain adequate emotional support for patient and others close to the patient

Assist the terminally ill patient to complete unfinished tasks and achieve a dignified death

### Hygiene and General Precautions

A question often asked by AIDS patients is how to decrease the chance of contracting opportunistic infections. Many organisms capable of causing infection in an immunosuppressed person are common in the environment, so exposure cannot be entirely avoided. However, good hygiene can reduce the risk. Since hand-to-mouth transmission of infectious material is extremely common, frequent handwashing with antimicrobial soap is the most basic and effective means of preventing infection, especially after using the bathroom and after handling pets, raw foods, soil, or houseplants. The risk of infection can also be reduced by avoiding places containing decaying vegetation, pigeon or other bird droppings, or accumulations of dust, since these are sites known to harbor fungal and bacterial organisms. Also, the patients should not travel to geographic areas where amebic or protozoal infections are endemic.

Within the home, normal house cleaning is usually adequate, but specific recommendations to inhibit the growth of microorganisms include disinfection of the bathroom with household bleach, frequent cleaning of air-conditioning filters, and periodic cleaning of aerators on water faucets. Food should be properly prepared to avoid or kill infectious organisms. Meats should be well cooked, and uncooked or commercially prepared meats should not be eaten. Raw fruits and vegetables should be peeled or carefully washed before being eaten. No eating utensils or drinking glasses should be shared.

Adequate nutrition at home helps to bolster resistance to infection. Frequent high calorie and protein snacks should be added to the diet. Meals should be balanced, with calories added through the use of such things as cream- or egg-based sauces, cheeses, milk powder, and grains. Fad diets, such as those based on macrobiotics, are frequently unbalanced and have not been demonstrated to be of significant worth.

Because of their immune defect, AIDS patients must avoid prolonged or intimate contact with people known to have infections, viral illnesses, coldlike symptoms, or draining lesions, and should stay away from crowds and crowded rooms. However, remaining totally housebound, without social contact or stimulation, is not advisable since this would only contribute to the sense of isolation that so often accompanies AIDS.

Sexual activity raises a practical, moral, and ethical dilemma for AIDS victims that they must resolve without evading the knowledge that intercourse may not only transmit their disease but also expose them to other serious sexually transmitted infections. If a decision is made to engage in sexual activity, AIDS patients and partners would be well-advised to avoid direct oral or rectal contact and to use a condom.

The AIDS patient at home often has fears about transmitting AIDS to other household members. Friends or family involved in caring for the patient may have ambivalent feelings about their risk of exposure that they are reluctant to express. Professional assistance with home care can provide an opportunity for patient and family to explore these fears in a reassuring environment and to be given information necessary to alleviate inappropriate concerns. For example, in addition to the known facts about how AIDS is transmitted, they should be told that no health-care workers involved in the care of AIDS patients have contracted the disease. Precautions to prevent exposure to the patient's blood and body fluids are similar to those employed in the hospital, as detailed in Chapter 14.

**Home-Care Skills**

People in the home often worry about their ability to provide adequate care and comfort to the physicially dependent patient. The skills required for home care may include bathing, positioning and turning the patient in bed, helping with walking, feeding, making the patient comfortable, and some specialized skills such as changing dressings. Many of these skills can be demonstrated for home care providers under professional guidance while the patient is still hospitalized. Visiting nurses and home health aides can provide and demonstrate the skills in the home. Also, in most cities, home-care courses are available through community service agencies, in some

## SUMMARY

AIDS patients have many care needs similar to those of other seriously ill persons. However, unique aspects of this disease, such as its transmissibility and association with specific groups in the population, require heightened awareness and sensitivity on the part of care providers. Whether care is provided by skilled professionals in the hospital or by family and friends at home, the common goal is to care about the AIDS patients as an individual and to communicate that caring through their actions.

# 14 Preventing AIDS

## JOHN W. SENSAKOVIC AND BENJAMIN GREER

In a dimly lit isolation room in a local medical center, an 18-year-old girl battles for her life against a severe and unusual pneumonia. The girl is an AIDS patient, her illness apparently acquired from her 20-year-old boyfriend, an intravenous-drug abuser previously afflicted with AIDS. The girl will not survive despite the expertise of a team of infectious-disease experts. The problem will not end here. The following day, a hospital employee will be suspended for refusing to enter the room in which the girl was treated. A local policeman will be suspended for refusing to transport the boyfriend after arrest on a drug charge. The girl's family will not only be distraught over the loss of their daughter, but greatly concerned for their own health and that of their other children. The funeral director will express anxiety about preparing the body and reluctance to open the casket for viewing due to his fear of AIDS.

This sequence of events is not all all unusual. Every case of AIDS involves many individuals who dread contracting the devastating illness. This paralyzing fear is not surprising since AIDS has received so much media attention and scientific knowledge is still lacking about many aspects of the disease. Unfortunately, the fear is all too often out of proportion to the scientific facts that are known about the transmission of AIDS. This chapter will discuss these facts, realistic precautions that should be taken, and unrealistic fears that should be avoided.

## PRECAUTIONS FOR HEALTH-CARE PERSONNEL

Members of the health-care profession, by the nature of their work, are continuously exposed to diseases, many serious or even fatal. This entails a risk they are aware of from the moment they enter the profession, and, to some extent, it is a risk they are expected to accept. At the same time, it is no less expected that the scientific community and regulating agencies will protect these professionals, wherever possible, from undue risks of such infection. It would be unprofessional and unacceptable for any health-care professional to refuse to care for any patient because of a possible inherent risk of infection. Likewise, it would be unacceptable for the scientific community and regulating agencies to allow such a risk to exceed the currently accepted minimal level of safety. It is the purpose of this section to review currently accepted precautions for minimizing the risk that health care professionals will contract AIDS.

Available information suggests that the transmission of AIDS resembles that of the hepatitis B virus: by blood, blood products, body secretions such as saliva, and excretions such as urine and feces. All major precautions against the transmission of AIDS are directed against contamination with these substances, as is done with hepatitis B-infected patients.

Since blood is thought to be one of the potentially most infectious vehicles for AIDS, most precautions aim to prevent contact with the blood of known or suspected AIDS patients. For health-care workers in particular, contact with the blood of an AIDS victim is thought to be the most serious risk and must be avoided. In particular, extraordinary care should be taken to avoid being accidentally stuck by a contaminated needle, cut by a surgical instrument, or splashed by contaminated blood on an open cut or wound. This risk is especially great for physicians, nurses, personnel who draw blood, and laboratory technicians who test blood. Gloves should always be worn when handling AIDS blood specimens and objects exposed to the blood of AIDS patients. Gowns should be worn when clothing may be soiled with blood, and hands should be washed immediately and thoroughly after contact with the blood of an AIDS patient. Blood specimens from AIDS patients should always be labeled as such, and accidental spills should be cleaned up promptly with a disinfectant solution such as household bleach. Contaminated articles should be placed in a leakproof bag and labeled before sterilization or incineration. All instruments used on AIDS patients should be properly sterilized before reuse.

Needle-stick injuries undoubtedly present one of the greatest risks of infection for health-care personnel. They are often due to lack of attention to the procedure and generally occur when the needle cover is replaced over the needle. Utmost attention must be paid to any procedure involving use of a needle. Gloves should be worn when blood is being drawn. Needles should not be reinserted into the needle cover, but placed directly into a puncture-resistant, disposable container; they should not be broken prior to disposal to prevent the splashing of possibly infectious blood.

Other body fluids and excretions from AIDS patients, such as saliva, tears, urine, and feces, are also considered to be possibly infectious, although probably less so than blood. These materials should be handled with the same precautions recommended for blood. Isolation procedures for AIDS are a recurrent concern for hospital personnel and administrators alike. Following the example of hepatitis B, currently recommended isolation procedures are designed to prevent exposure to AIDS patients' blood, secretions, and excretions. A private room is probably desirable, if for no other reason than to act as a reminder of the importance of isolation techniques. If the patient is unable to maintain good hygiene, a private room is mandatory. Gowns, gloves, and scrupulous hand washing are essential. Masks are not necessary, unless there is a possibility that the patient's saliva will be sprayed into the air, as frequently happens when a patient on a ventilator is suctioned. When there is any risk of the spraying or splashing of infectious materials, protective eye coverings should also be used.

Recommended precautions for hospital and laboratory personnel are outlined in tables 1 and 2. They are appropriate and reasonable. If carefully followed, they assure a minimal risk for health-care personnel responsible for the treatment of AIDS patients. Using these precautions as a guide also forestalls the addition of unrealistic and unnecessary procedures that can often increase anxiety in caring for

## TABLE 1.   PRECAUTIONS FOR HOSPITAL PERSONNEL TREATING POSSIBLE AIDS PATIENTS

Avoid wounds with contaminated needles or instruments.
Avoid contact of open wounds with contaminated materials.
Wear gloves.
Wear gowns.
Wash hands thoroughly.
Label contaminated specimens and materials.
Transport contaminated items in impervious bags.
Clean spills quickly with bleach.
Do not break needles.
(From *Morbidity and Mortality Weekly Reports*, 31:577–579, 1982.)


## TABLE 2.   PRECAUTIONS FOR LABORATORY PERSONNEL PERFORMING TESTS ON MATERIALS FROM POSSIBLE AIDS PATIENTS

Do not pipet by mouth.
Dispose of needles properly.
Wear lab coats.
Wear gloves.
Wash hands thoroughly.
Disinfect work area with bleach.
(From *Morbidity and Mortality Weekly Reports*, 31:577–579, 1982.)


AIDS patients and sometimes even prevent providing the optimal medical care they so often desperately need.

## PRECAUTIONS FOR AIDS PATIENTS, RISK GROUPS, AND CLOSE CONTACTS

The scientific community has defined well the AIDS risks and precautions for health-care personnel, who are unavoidably exposed by occupation. It has not adequately informed the general public, for most of whom the risks are exceedingly small. No doubt this is partly due to the difficulty for scientists to downplay a problem treated with such sensationalism by the media.

By far, the greatest risk of AIDS is found in the homosexual and drug-addict populations. Their risk is specifically associated with close sexual contact or the injection of drugs into the body. The rest of the general population is not at significant risk.

Measures can be taken to minimize the threat of AIDS. The maintenance of sound general health is the mainstay against any infectious disease. Substance abuse of any kind is dangerous and may reduce the body's ability to defend itself against infectious agents. Intravenous-drug abuse is particularly dangerous, because the common practice of sharing syringes and needles provides the avenue for direct transmission of the infectious agent responsible for AIDS from one person to another.

Maintenance of good health means following sensible guidelines, including regular health checkups by a physician, eating a well-balanced diet, and the control of any diseases requiring medical supervision. People who have unexplained fevers, gland swellings, skin rashes, diarrhea, weight loss, or a persistent cough should seek medical advice to determine the cause of what may be more than just persistent and annoying symptoms.

Transmission of AIDS by sexual contact causes an important concern. While the number of AIDS cases does not indicate a threat of the order of herpes disease and gonorrhea, AIDS is often fatal and has no known cure. Although the homosexual population is a main risk group, to say that AIDS is just a homosexual disease is wrong, for several cases have resulted from heterosexual contact. Avoidance of sex with partners of whom little is known, particularly with regard to general health, is of utmost importance. In addition, the risk of AIDS rises with increases in the number of sexual partners per year. However, knowing that a sexual partner is now in good health and not promiscuous is no guarantee of complete safety, primarily because a person who has contracted AIDS may not show the initial symptoms for as much as 6 months to 2 years later. During this incubation period, the potential for contagion is uncertain. Moreover, the ability of a physician to diagnose AIDS during this time is difficult because symptoms may be few and nonspecific.

Rumors of contracting AIDS by casual contact with an AIDS patient, or with an object touched by an AIDS patient, have no basis in fact. Many other unfounded fears must also be dispelled. For example, some prospective blood donors have been disturbed by a rumor that AIDS can somehow be spread through blood-drawing equipment. The truth is that equipment is sterile and not reused, so that giving blood incurs no risk of contracting AIDS.

Blood transfusion is a different matter. The risk comes from receiving blood that may theoretically be carrying the AIDS agent. This risk is difficult to calculate but is extremely small in most situations, and is outweighed by the benefits of receiving urgently needed blood. Patients with diseases that necessitate frequent blood transfusions, such as hemophiliacs and people with sickle-cell disease, may face a greater theoretical risk because of increased exposure. Again, the risk is heavily outweighed by the need for the blood products being received. It has been suggested that the risk for hemophiliacs can be reduced by substituting the cryoprecipitate for the more commonly used commercial Factor-VIII freeze-dried concentrate. The reason given is that the cryoprecipitate is obtained from plasma of only one blood donor, while Factor-VIII concentrate comes from a plasma pool involving thousands of donors. In either case, it cannot be overemphasized that, when the need for blood products is indicated, the benefits of transfusion are high, and the risks from not receiving needed blood are far greater than the theoretical risks of contracting AIDS via the transfusion.

Transmission of AIDS by means other than intimate sexual contact and transfusion of blood products is, at most, unlikely. No one has yet reported an airborne source of AIDS, nor have doctors who treat many AIDS patients contracted the disease. It therefore seems reasonably certain that one cannot contract AIDS by being in the same room or shaking hands with an AIDS patient, or from a toilet seat used by a patient. Transmission of AIDS requires frequent and intimate contact.

Several professions have duties that may involve contact with AIDS victims. For example, firemen and first-aid personnel are concerned about the possibility of contracting AIDS from transporting patients or administering cardiopulmonary resuscitation (CPR). Casual contact in transportation carries no risk. The question of CPR is not so simple, since contact with saliva or blood in the mouth during mouth-to-mouth resuscitation may pose some risk. Hence, direct mouth-to-mouth resuscitation should be avoided with known AIDS patients, but should never be denied to a patient with an unknown history.

Police and corrections officers worry about contact with prisoners, a group known to have a high incidence of drug abuse and homosexuality. Again, casual contact incurs no risk, but bites or other exposure to blood, excretions, or saliva, that may result from confrontations in correctional systems, should be avoided if possible. Exposure should be followed by thorough washing and disinfection. In our experience, a three-pronged educational and screening program alleviates fear of AIDS among prison workers and assures them that their risk is minimal. The program involves providing AIDS facts to corrections officers, inmates, and the institutional health service and screening for AIDS among inmates.

Placement of AIDS patients after release from the hospital is one of the most difficult problems in AIDS management. Anxiety among the patient's family members can be devastating, as illustrated by a recent case. Two young sisters were diagnosed as having contracted AIDS through drug usage. Both were hospitalized for a long time and had a complicated illness. Family members frequently visited the hospital and were obviously concerned, especially when the survival of both girls was in doubt. When the girls did improve, they were taken home, only to be brought back to the hospital emergency room two days later and abandoned by the family with only the hospital gowns they wore when they were discharged.

This reaction is not unusual. The family is concerned for their own safety and have many questions. Where should the patient sleep, wash, eat? How should clothes, dishes, utensils, and bedroom be cleaned? The questions are reasonable and must be answered to increase understanding and reduce unrealistic fears.

AIDS patients at home should have separate rooms and certainly their own beds. Contact by the family and visitors with soiled clothing and objects should be avoided, and gloves should be worn when handling them. Razors, shavers, and toothbrushes must not be shared, since they can become contaminated with minute amounts of blood. Special precautions for clothing, dishes, and disinfection are described in table 3. Since casual contact carries no risk, there is no

**TABLE 3.    PRECAUTIONS FOR AIDS PATIENTS AT HOME**

Necessary equipment:
  Thermometer
  Antimicrobial soap
  Household bleach solution (1 part bleach–10 parts water)
  Large and small plastic bags
  Garbage receptacles
  Gloves
  Paper towels
Precautions to be followed:
  Wear rubber gloves when handling contaminated and soiled articles.
  Wash hands with antimicrobial soap after handling contaminated
    and soiled articles.
  Place all contaminated articles in a tied plastic bag and discard bag
    in a large, lined garbage receptacle to be emptied daily.
  Wash all contaminated surfaces immediately. Wash bathroom sink,
    toilet, and bathtub daily with bleach solution.
  Soak all soiled clothing and linen in bleach solution in bathtub for
    1 hour before washing.
  Patients should have their own eating utensils, razor, shaver, and
    toothbrush stored separately in plastic bags.

reason that the AIDS patients cannot be returned home if these precautions are understood by patient and family. To achieve such understanding, the help of an experienced social worker and visiting
nurse can be extremely valuable.

## SUMMARY

Careful medical surveillance and screening are essential for AIDS
patients as well as members of high-risk groups. Activities known to
increase risk, such as multiple sexual partners and intravenous-drug
abuse must be avoided completely. In addition, it is now recommended that members of high-risk groups refrain from donating
blood or plasma. Maintenance of proper hygienic measures are mandatory to assure minimal risk to others. A well-balanced diet, with a

high caloric intake to prevent or minimize weight loss is essential. In addition to proper diet, adequate rest and avoidance of exposure to persons with contagious illness are necessary.

On the basis of available information, the preceding pages have outlined mandatory and reasonable AIDS precautions and attempted to separate them from foolish and unnecessary fears. Until the AIDS dilemma is solved, these precautions will assure minimal risk to society and maximal advantage to AIDS patients.

# 15      Psychological and Social Issues of AIDS and Strategies for Survival

## VIRGINIA LEHMAN AND NOREEN RUSSELL

The impact of AIDS is catastrophic for those it strikes, their families, and their friends. This chapter will highlight psychological and social aspects of AIDS and resources helpful in fighting the disease.

Many of the psychosocial aspects of AIDS are like those of other chronic and devastating illnesses. Individuals ". . . usually experience heightened states of anxiety, fear and depression induced by physical pain and psycho-social distress. A number of factors contribute to these emotions: imminent separation from all that is meaningful in life; treatment regimes of chemotherapy; experiences of physical deterioration . . . . These dysfunctional emotions reduce the ability of patients to cope with their difficult life situations" (Allison et al., 1983).

### FEARS OF CONTAGION

What further sets the AIDS patient apart is the unknown nature of the illness and the fear of contagion. Patients worry about transmitting AIDS to loved ones, and associates of AIDS patients are concerned about contracting the disease. Unanswered questions about the disease's infectious nature compound these concerns.

This fear is perhaps the most characteristic response to this illness. Most chronic-care hospitals and skilled nursing homes do not accept people with AIDS, and employers and landlords become alarmed upon learning that an employee or tenant has AIDS. The mother of one AIDS patient was reluctant to have her stricken daughter remain in the home; she feared that the illness might spread to the daughter's two children. A man threatened to remove his children from the household if his wife's brother, an AIDS patient, came to live with the family. Unfortunately, the fear some patients have of abandonment is sometimes borne out in reality.

AIDS patients' feelings of stigmatization are frequently underscored during hospitalization. Patients are often placed in isolation, and hospital staff and visitors are required to wear masks, gowns, and gloves. Some patients remain in hospital isolation for weeks. As each day passes, the AIDS patient feels more distant from the real world. This further intensifies a sense of not belonging, being different, being untouchable. Many patients liken this experience to being a leper.

AIDS patients are continuously concerned about contracting random infections because their defective immune systems make them less able to resist illness. Some patients fear and avoid public places where exposure to germs is greater.

## DEPENDENCY AND LOVE IN AIDS

On learning that they have AIDS, individuals react in a variety of ways. Some panic, others go into shock. It may take days or weeks for them to acknowledge the diagnosis. Some retreat into denial, consulting many different physicians in hope that the diagnosis was wrong. There is a sense of disbelief, anger, and self-blame.

Coping with a life-threatening illness is extremely stressful. AIDS victims are subject to repeated hospitalizations, each longer than the one before. Medical tests and treatment may sometimes be painful, and physicians differ over appropriate treatment, for example, chemotherapy versus interferon. Thus, patients and families must choose a form of medical treatment espoused by some physicians while discouraged by others. As the illness progresses and becomes more debilitating, both the patient and the family question whether they made the right choice. Because there is no definitive protocol, confidence and trust in one's doctor are especially important ingredients in fighting the disease.

Horror stories abound of AIDS patients being abandoned by hospital staff and others. They have been left unattended in hospital rooms, evicted from their homes, and terminated from jobs. However, these rejections are far outnumbered by stories in which family, friends, and lovers have demonstrated courageous devotion and care. Many have traveled long distances to be with the ill person, often at great sacrifice—leaving their own homes, their families, their towns for a strange city where services are unfamiliar.

Because AIDS predominantly affects young adults—people in their late twenties, thirties, and forties—caretaking responsibilities are often thrust on elderly parents in their sixties and seventies. In our culture, the usual adult role is assisting and caring for elderly parents. The necessity for this sudden "role reversal" tends to create additional stress—the patient regresses not only because of illness, but because of forced dependency on an elderly parent. Patterns of relating as child to parent become more pronounced.

An energetic woman in her seventies, the mother of a young AIDS patient, resided in another city. On two separate occasions, she left behind the rest of her family and her job to care for her sick adult son. She prepared his favorite meals and performed all household chores. At times, tensions were strong. He felt that she was overly protective and constantly "chatting and moving about," while she felt he was insensitive and a bully. She remained with him until he died, often spending ten hours a day at the hospital. Similarly, the laborer father of another young man cared for his son around the clock. Although unaccustomed to bathing his son and changing bedpans, the father performed these tasks with loving devotion during the course of his son's terminal illness.

AIDS victims' lovers may be equally devoted. Stories of great attentiveness, sensitivity, and love are frequent. The homosexual lover, despite membership in a high-risk group, places loyalty to his ill mate above concern for personal safety. In many instances, an AIDS patient has been discharged to return home where his lover became his main caretaker, providing comfort and care until the patient died.

## GUILT AND SHAME

Self-condemnation is frequent among AIDS patients and close family members. This is particularly true of homosexual patients, who blame themselves for bringing on their illness. Conflicts about homosexuality surface. Feelings of discrimination, real and imagined, are common. For a troubled individual who has come to accept his homosexuality, the diagnosis of AIDS reawakens earlier ambivalence. Having attained a sense of freedom and pride in homosexuality, he may view AIDS as God's punishment for both his homosexuality and his pride. For those not "out of the closet," a diagnosis of AIDS may force the disclosure of their homosexuality. Family, employer, and even strangers become privy to what was private. Disclosure of homosexuality at a time of one's own choosing may no longer be an option.

Some families are unable to accept the fact that a son or brother is homosexual. Upon learning that a son had AIDS, one family told others that what he had was leukemia. They could talk to each other about his homosexuality, but felt ashamed with others. Another family feared what the neighbors might say and chose to keep the son's illness secret. Families have withdrawn from friends and neighbors in shame and fear of discrimination, thus denying themselves important sources of emotional support. Parents often blame themselves for their child's illness, agonizing whether they played a role in their son's homosexuality. There is also an assumed natural order of life, and parents do not expect their children to die before them.

## AIDS AND SEXUALITY

AIDS victims have a double sexual concern. By engaging in sex, they may transmit their disease to a lover and, because of their immunodeficiency, they may contract sexually transmitted infections that would further compromise their own health. Some patients lose interest in sexual activity, due to either a general lack of energy or fear of possible negative consequences. Many abstain out of moral concern about spreading the disease, even if sexual desire persists. For those used to a very active sexual life, abstinence also represents the loss of an entire social support network. This is particularly true for homosexuals accustomed to a "fast lifestyle" of bars, bathhouses, and anonymous sex.

Those in monogamous relationships are confronted with particularly poignant choices. Tension invariably develops over whether to have sex and which sexual activities are safe, and anxieties arise about the safety and health of the other.

## DEPENDENCY

Patients in later stages of AIDS need assistance with everyday activities. Some resist all support. One would not even allow friends to help with shopping and cleaning. His determination to go to the supermarket and bank himself and to clean his own apartment represented his mastery over illness. Completion of even one small household task was exhilarating. Others may accept help from family and friends, but continue struggling to maintain their independence. Still others feel, at times unrealistically, that they are helpless and expect others to do everything for them.

The personality of an individual predetermines how he or she will respond to illness. People who were independent and grasped initiatives before becoming ill continue to strive for independence afterward. Those who were dependent and expected that others would always care for them remain in that mold. A freelance graphic designer exemplified the independent's response to illness. He actively explored treatment options with his physician and kept himself informed at all times. In contrast, another AIDS patient had always felt that life was unfair and that others failed to accommodate his needs; after becoming ill, he made extraordinary and unrealistic demands on his friends. Family and friends relate and respond to sick loved ones much as they did before the onset of illness. Those with close ties maintain those ties; those with few friends or unsteady relationships may become isolated.

Feelings of anger and guilt affect both the ill person and the caretaker. The person who is ill feels anger at the affliction and guilt for being a burden. Family and friends feel guilty both for being well and for resenting the needs of the one who is ill. It is important for family members, friends, and lovers to turn away periodically from caretaking and have time for themselves. This serves as a safety valve to release tension. It also helps the ill person feel less guilty about being a burden.

When AIDS strikes, work and personal aspirations are put aside in the battle to survive. There is often a conflict between pursuing work and activity at as high a level as possible and slowing down and allowing others to help. Specific circumstances may determine the benefit of one approach over the other. For example, the manager of an antiques store, despite nausea and diarrhea, went to work every day. He took great pride in his store, and his love for his job kept him going. Another AIDS victim, with a more physically demanding job, found that he was no longer able to work. Despite much frustration and sadness, he yielded to his undeniable disability and accepted "being pampered." He had always been very helpful and giving to others; now he allowed others to be helpful and giving to him in his need.

## REACTIONS TO DEATH

R. Kastenbaum (Kastenbaum, 1977) coined the phrase "bereavement overload," referring to elderly individuals who experience the deaths of many friends within a relatively short period of time. A similar phenomenon is seen with AIDS: young adults are experiencing the loss of many friends within a few months or years. This is particularly devastating and frightening within the homosexual community.

Kubler-Ross describes death as ". . . a fearful, frightening happening . . . even if we think we have mastered it on many levels" (Kubler-Ross, 1969). Despite this natural fear, many individuals are able to talk about the fact that they are dying and put their affairs in order. Many specify the funeral service they prefer, whether they wish to be buried or cremated, and, if cremated, where their ashes are to be strewn. Many draw up wills for the first time. A quiet strength and determination are often present. Conflicts with loved ones are sometimes resolved. In one case, a man who had long been estranged from his family met with them the day before he died. They openly discussed differences, apologized for hurtful actions, and expressed their deep love for one another. This man achieved some final measure of equanimity. Despite the implications of terminal illness, AIDS victims usually want to live and fight for their survival.

## SURVIVAL STRATEGIES

Knowledge about entitlements and community resources can fortify patients in the face of illness. Eligibility requirements for these entitlements vary from state to state. The following are a list and general description of entitlement programs and community resources.

### Financial and Other Entitlements

*Public Assistance*

If you have AIDS, are unable to work, and are without financial assets, you may be eligible for public assistance. Apply at the nearest local or county welfare agency. Needed are documents that establish citizenship or legal alien status (e.g., birth certificate, baptismal record, alien registration green card), records of how you maintained yourself financially in the past year (rent receipts, paycheck stubs, copy of income tax return, telephone, gas, and electric bills sent to your address). You will also need a detailed letter from your physician or local hospital stating that you have an illness that prohibits you from working either full time or part time for at least one year. In many states, you must also apply for Supplemental Social Security (SSI) at the same time that you apply for public assistance (see Social Security below).

*Food Stamps*

Depending upon your financial status, you may be eligible for food stamps. Check with your local social service department.

*Disability Programs*

State

Many states have a disability program to which your employer may be contributing. However, if the company where you work has only a few employees, it may not be covered under this program. Your company's personnel staff can tell you if you are eligible and assist you with the necessary forms.

cases specifically for the care of AIDS patients. Further information about these courses may be obtained by calling one of the resource groups listed in Chapter 17.

### Emotional Stress

At home, as in the hospital, the AIDS patient needs emotional support. Family and friends are the patient's major source of emotional support, but participation in a community-based support group can add the needed perspective of a peer group. When group participation is not possible, many AIDS-related organizations will provide counselors who visit the home.

An often neglected aspect of home care is the stress imposed on the care giver. Tending to a sick loved one is a physically and emotionally demanding tast. After a time, the most devoted care giver may feel trapped by circumstances, frightened, exhausted, and frustrated or angry with the patient. While these feelings are natural and understandable, they may be difficult to accept and can induce guilt, especially if inappropriately expressed. Family and friends should be encouraged to take time off for themselves and to seek relief either from support groups or from relatives or acquaintances who will occasionally take turns caring for the AIDS patient.

AIDS is still a disease with no known cure. Patients must at some point face the fact that death may not be far off. Many find that planning for the terminal phase of illness alleviates some of the fears and anxiety that surround it. One issue for both the patient and loved ones is the extent of medical intervention desired when death appears imminent. Some may prefer to die at home without being subjected to life-prolonging measures and machinery. Others may elect hospitalization and various degrees of care. The wishes of patient and family should be thoroughly discussed in advance with the primary physician so that the limits of desired treatment are understood. Home-care providers may also find themselves assisting the patient to complete unfinished final tasks, such as arranging for the disposal of property and possessions, resolving conflicts with estranged family members, and specifying funeral rites. Doing whatever has to be done while there is still time insures that the patient's wishes will be carried out and often provides a degree of comfort in the final days of the illness.

### Social Security

The Social Security Administration has two disability programs, Social Security Disability (SSD) and Supplemental Social Security (SSI). A diagnosis of AIDS, as specified by the Centers for Disease Control, establishes your disability. If you have contributed to Social Security through employment and have worked the required length of time, you most likely are eligible for Social Security disability. Benefits are based solely on your prior participation in the system and proof that you have AIDS. Eligibility for SSI is based on disability plus lack of financial resources. For either program, you apply at the nearest Social Security office where the staff are very helpful and will inform you about both programs. You will need documents to prove citizenship or legal alien status and a letter from your doctor or hospital stating specifically that you have AIDS and are unable to work full time or part time for at least one year.

### Veterans Administration Benefits

If you served in the armed forces during wartime, were honorably discharged, and can present proof of a permanent and total disability, you may be eligible for a VA disability pension. Check with your local VA office for information and forms.

### Union Benefits

If you belong to a union, check with your representative about eligibility for disability programs.

## Health Insurance

### Individual or Group Health Insurance

It is important to check what services are covered under your policy. Some policies are comprehensive and others are not. You may wish to supplement the coverage of your present policy. Contact your insurance company with questions about your current policy and possibly desirable additional riders. It is a good idea to check with several companies and compare policies and costs.

### Government

Most states provide some medical coverage to individuals with limited financial assets and no medical insurance. Proof of citizenship, legal residency, and financial documents are necessary to establish eligibility. In many states, this program covers a wide range of medical services, e.g., homemaker help and medical equipment. Local hospitals and social service departments can provide specific application information.

*Veterans Administration*

If you are a veteran with an honorable discharge, you can obtain medical care at the nearest VA hospital/clinic. Except in acute medical emergencies, veterans with service-connected disabilities are given preference.

**Legal Matters**

Having a will is very important. Not only does a will provide for the disposal of your property as you would wish, but it also protects your heirs. The state receives a disproportionate amount of your money if you die without having a will. A will insures a more prompt estate settlement and also conveys your preference regarding burial or cremation.

A power of attorney may be necessary if there is no next of kin. This can have special significance if the dying person is confused and unable to make necessary decisions. Mental confusion is not uncommon in AIDS, especially in the later stages of the illness. A durable power of attorney is the most comprehensive, since it does not have to be periodically renewed. Assigning a power of attorney to a trusted friend can facilitate the rendering of appropriate medical treatment and assist with many practical details.

Some hospitals do not recognize the partner in homosexual relationships as equivalent to a spouse or relative; parents or siblings, rather than a person's lover, may be called upon to render important decisions. In such cases, a power of attorney will not empower a lover to make decisions if there is a next of kin. Make sure to familiarize yourself with your hospital's practices in this respect. It is also recommended that the AIDS patient, lover, and family discuss and understand the patient's wishes to avoid painful and unnecessary conflict.

## Community Resources

### Hospitals

Teaching hospitals, especially in major cities, have medical staff experienced in treating AIDS patients. Inquire at your local hospital if any members of the staff are specially trained to treat AIDS. Many hospitals offer crisis intervention services as well as individual, family, and group therapy. The staffs of hospitals that receive federal funding have at least one trained social worker who is knowledgeable about community resources and entitlement programs and will be able to assist you.

### Psychotherapy/Counseling Services

Crisis intervention involves on-the-spot telephone and in-person counseling. Counseling can be vitally important to AIDS victims and their families. Hospitals, mental health clinics, and special AIDS support programs offer this service. Some churches and synagogues also offer counseling services in addition to pastoral care.

Psychotherapy can accommodate the individual, the family unit, and groups of individuals with common concerns. Therapeutic approaches vary with the training of the therapist and the orientation of the clinic. The most effective type of psychotherapeutic counseling depends upon the needs and circumstances of the patient and family. Psychotherapy services are available through hospitals, clinics, specialized agencies, and private practitioners. Before choosing, request information about staff credentials and the cost of services.

Agencies developed in response to AIDS, such as the Gay Men's Health Crisis and the AIDS Resource Center in New York City, and Shanti in San Francisco, can refer you to experienced practitioners. Groups such as the American Psychiatric Association, the American Psychological Association, the Society of Clinical Social Work Psychotherapists, and gay and lesbian clinical psychotherapy associations may also be good sources of referrals.

Funeral directors are another source of assistance to the families and friends of AIDS patients. It is helpful to obtain advance information about burial and cremation procedures and costs. Your state funeral directors' association can help you to obtain this information.

### Home Health Agencies

Home health agencies provide services in the home. Every state has a visiting nurse service. At the request of a physician, a nurse will assess the patient's health needs and offer skilled nursing care in the home. The service may also provide homemakers, home health attendants, social workers, and physical therapists. Homemakers assist with shopping and light housekeeping; home health attendants assist with bathing and personal care of patients in addition to household chores. In large cities, public and private agencies offer in-home health-support services. Some agencies have staff especially trained to assist with AIDS patients.

The American Red Cross of Greater New York offers a training program for family and friends of AIDS patients entitled "Home Nursing for AIDS Care Givers." The course covers basic skills and information necessary for the appropriate care of homebound AIDS patients. It also teaches precautions to control the spread of the disease.

### Specialized Agencies

#### Cancer

For AIDS patients who have cancer, agencies such as the American Cancer Society and Cancer Care are a source of special help. Help ranges from homemaker services to payment of some of the costs of transportation for hospital visits and the purchase of medical equipment. Cancer Care also offers both individual and group counseling.

#### Gay Men's Health Crisis, New York City

The need for a special group to deal with the AIDS crisis became clear at a meeting in August 1981 where Dr. Alvin E. Friedman-Kien spoke to a group of about 80 men. Dr. Friedman-Kien had been credited with citing new cases of Kaposi's sarcoma as an unprecedented outbreak of an old disease in a new context—among formerly healthy, relatively young, gay men. It was suggested at the meeting that a group be formed to raise money for medical research. That group became formally known as the Gay Men's Health Crisis (GMHC).

As the needs of AIDS patients grew, GMHC expanded its purpose and services. It is now a nonprofit organization with 11 full-time and 3 part-time employees, and over 1,100 volunteers. Its structure is open and fluid, with no exclusionary rules and no requirements for membership other than a genuine concern about the health of gay men.

In addition to funding medical research projects, GMHC provides a full range of clinical and educational services. All prospective patients who contact GMHC for help are visited within 24 hours by a licensed mental-health professional from the admissions division. A comprehensive, psychosocial, intake interview is conducted, and a report is written with recommendations for treatment and referral to one or more GMHC services, including crisis intervention counseling, a buddy support service, patient recreation services, an AIDS self-help support group, an AIDS therapy group, a care partner therapy group, a women's support group, financial counseling services, and individual psychotherapy services.

In an extensive effort to provide accurate, up-to-date information and advice about AIDS to the general public and to special high-risk populations, GMHC has undertaken a number of educational activities. It regularly holds public forums and training seminars, operates an around-the-clock AIDS hotline, provides technical assistance to volunteer organizations similar to GMHC, distributes newsletters and brochures, and maintains an archive of published information on AIDS.

### AIDS Resource Center (ARC), New York City

The AIDS Resource Center (ARC) was founded in February 1983 by a group of concerned persons who had had direct experience with the death of a friend or lover afflicted with AIDS. ARC coordinated its activities with GMHC to fill gaps in service, particularly in the areas of housing, direct financial assistance, and spiritual support.

ARC developed short- and long-term housing resources for AIDS patients with the overall goal of establishing hospice-like facilities. The ARC staff is actively engaged in locating a suitable building to be used as a hospice.

AIDS patients may receive direct financial aid, as a grant or loan, up to a maximum of $500 per individual and are encouraged to apply for loans. At times, recipients of aid repay ARC in kind, e.g., by doing clerical work or manning the telephone.

The spiritual support rendered by this agency is unique. Weekend retreats for patients and close associates are held in a scenic, secluded area of Connecticut. The holistic approach encompasses Christian worship, nutrition, exercise, and meditation. Participation in programs is voluntary, and scholarships are available for those unable to pay.

Group therapy at ARC differs from that at other agencies in the use of prayer as the primary source of solace. ARC also offers bereavement counseling, in both individual and group sessions.

Formal spiritual counseling is an integral part of ARC's program. All major religious groups are represented, including all Protestant denominations, all three divisions of the Hebrew faith, Muslims, and various sects. ARC is preparing an educational packet about AIDS for distribution to all churches in the metropolitian New York area.

ARC also sponsors a hospital visit program in cooperation with the Volunteer and Social Work Departments at Bellevue Hospital Center, New York City. Bellevue volunteers undergo basic training in working with acutely ill people, addressing spiritual needs, and using community resources. This program was developed to supplement the CMHC buddy system. The volunteers visit AIDS patients only in the hospital and cooperate with the hospital social work staff in providing appropriate service.

*Shanti Project, San Francisco*

The Shanti (Sanskrit for "inner peace") Project, also a nonprofit organization, was founded in 1974 by Dr. Charles Garfield to provide free volunteer counseling services in the San Francisco Bay area to individuals and families facing a life-threatening illness and bereavement. Volunteers are carefully screened, receive extensive training and continuing supervision, and attend weekly support group meetings.

Shanti Project contracted with the San Francisco Department of Public Health to provide supportive services to the community made necessary by the AIDS epidemic. In addition to financial support from the City and County of San Francisco, funding comes from foundations and individual contributions.

Services of the Shanti Project include:

Individual Counseling—Volunteer counselors work on a one-to-one basis with AIDS patients and their loved ones and are available for short or long terms according to individual needs. A Shanti volunteer will make home or hospital visits.

Support Groups—Ongoing support groups are offered for AIDS patients, individuals with chronic AIDS-like symptoms, and lovers, family, and friends of AIDS patients.

Community Volunteer Program—Shanti volunteers help with the practical problems of AIDS patients, running errands, arranging transportation, grocery shopping, preparing meals, housecleaning, etc.

Shanti Project Residence Program—Long-term, low-cost housing is provided for AIDS patients with housing problems. Specific requirements for eligibility include details such as: 3-month previous residence in San Francisco, medical diagnosis of AIDS, financial need, displacement from previous residence, and ability and willingness to participate in the housing program. Application involves filling out forms to establish eligibility requirements and an interview with the Residence Director. Placement depends upon available vacancies. Assistance in finding interim housing is given through the Shanti Residence office, the AIDS/KS Foundation, and the City of San Francisco. Since eligibility requirements are subject to change, individuals interested in the program should contact the Shanti Project directly.

Newsletter—A monthly newsletter is available to AIDS patients. It contains such information as services offered at low or no cost, educational and social meetings and activities, medical updates, and alternative forms of therapy.

Counseling at San Francisco General Hospital—Through a special contract with the hospital, Shanti provides counselors for an inpatient unit and an outpatient clinic. Both individual counseling and continuing support groups are available for patients, lovers, families, and friends.

Training and Educational Seminars—The Shanti Project conducts general seminars for the public and professionals involved in the care of the ill and the bereaved. Special programs are available to social service agencies, health-care institutions, counselors, clergy, universities, and the general public. Shanti also provides consultation for groups that want to establish services in their own communities.

\* \* \*

Shanti requires direct contact from anyone requesting counseling service unless physical circumstances make it impossible. The telephone number is (415) 588-9644, and the mailing address is 890 Hayes Street, San Francisco, CA 94117.

## SUMMARY

AIDS patients are forced to make many difficult psychological and social adjustments. They are faced with painful illness and treatment, possible loss of job and income, loss of independence, and a reassessment of social and personal needs. Relationships change—some become strained, others develop into deep, supportive, meaningful ties. It is essential that patients, family, and friends avail themselves of the psychological and social support of the community. Various sources of help are available.

# 16    Questions and Answers about AIDS

## MICHAEL MARSH, VICTOR GONG,
## AND DANIEL SHINDLER

**WHAT IS AIDS?**

AIDS is an impairment of the body's ability to fight disease. It is acquired, meaning that it is neither inherited nor a genetic condition. The disease depresses the body's immune system, leaving the individual vulnerable to a wide spectrum of opportunistic infections and malignancies. Because of the large number of characteristic signs and symptoms that define this disorder, AIDS is called a syndrome, that is, a collection of many different symptoms appearing together.

The most common opportunistic infections of AIDS patients are *Pneumocystis carinii* pneumonia and Kaposi's sarcoma, although many other infections may appear in sequence or simultaneously, over the course of the disease.

Defining AIDS is difficult because clinicians and researchers have not agreed on standardized criteria to characterize the syndrome and its diagnosis. There is no definitive test that can confirm a diagnosis of AIDS. However, the Centers for Disease Control (CDC) has proposed certain strict guidelines that most physicians apply in making the diagnosis. According to CDC guidelines, AIDS should be suspected in any person who is under the age of 60, develops opportunistic infections and malignancies, is a member of one of the known risk groups for AIDS, and shows laboratory evidence of impaired cellular immunity. However, milder forms of AIDS-related illnesses may be overlooked by these guidelines. The full spectrum of AIDS-related illnesses is unknown, but is thought to include the lymphade-nopathy syndrome (swollen glands), autoimmune disorders, and the wasting syndrome.

Thus, AIDS can be characterized as a syndrome with a broad clinical spectrum, ranging from severe infections and death to asymp-tomatic disease (e.g., carriers and patients who have recovered), in-cluding milder forms with perhaps a better prognosis than overt AIDS.

## WHO IS AT RISK?

The first cases of AIDS in the United States were gay men. Since then, other population groups found to be at high risk include:

Bisexual or gay men sexually active with many different male partners
Intravenous-drug abusers who share needles
Immigrant and native Haitians
Hemophiliacs and others who require transfusions of large amounts of blood and blood products
Heterosexual partners of AIDS patients
Infants and children of high-risk parents

## WHAT ARE THE SYMPTOMS OF AIDS?

Symptoms may be totally nonspecific. No characteristic symptoms clearly establish the diagnosis of AIDS. In its mildest forms, AIDS may even go unnoticed. In severe cases, symptoms may develop and progress very rapidly. The symptoms may include:

Swollen glands, usually in the neck, armpit, or groin, with or with-out pain
Unexpected weight loss, usually 10–15 pounds or more in 2 months, not due to deliberate dieting
A persistent cough and shortness of breath not related to a "flu" or cigarette smoking
Purple or pink bumps under the skin or in the mouth, nose, and rectum, looking like bruises that don't go away

Persistent fever for over 1–2 weeks

Night sweats—waking up at night drenched in perspiration, persisting for several weeks

Persistent diarrhea not explainable by diet or a "stomach virus"

A thick, whitish coating on the tongue and/or the mouth, with or without a sore throat

## WHAT IS AN OPPORTUNISTIC INFECTION?

Without normal immune function, the body is vulnerable to assault by many environmental toxins and pathogens. An opportunistic infection is one that does not usually arise in a healthy person with a sound immune system, but strikes where a microorganism finds an immune system that is defective. For example, all of us have potentially toxic viruses, bacteria, yeasts, and possibly cancer cells in our bodies. They do us no harm because a normal immune surveillance system keeps them in check. However, if the body's immune defenses are diminished for any reason, these pathogens have the opportunity to flourish and create infection. Thus, a local yeast infection can grow and swarm throughout the body, and the previously rare and nonaggressive *Pneumocystis carinii* can cause a severe pneumonia.

## WHAT IS *PNEUMOCYSTIS CARINII* PNEUMONIA?

*Pneumocystis carinii* pneumonia (PCP) is the most common disease in AIDS. It is due to a parasite and is characterized by fever, a nonproductive cough, weight loss, drenching night sweats, and shortness of breath. Before AIDS was recognized, PCP was seen only rarely, in premature infants, debilitated children and adults, and in patients whose immunologic responses are suppressed by chemotherapy or to prevent rejection of a transplanted organ. With the advent of AIDS, the number of cases has increased dramatically. Unfortunately, the underlying immune dysfunction hinders recovery from PCP, and it is the leading cause of death in AIDS patients.

## WHAT IS KAPOSI'S SARCOMA?

After PCP, Kaposi's sarcoma (KS) is the second most common disease associated with AIDS, afflicting over a third of all AIDS patients. KS is a rare malignant skin tumor that, before 1979, affected elderly men of Mediterranean descent. Typically, it was limited to the skin, rarely affected other organs, and responsed well to treatment. Patients often lived for 8 to 13 years after diagnosis and usually died of other diseases related to old age.

Another variety of KS is found in equatorial Africa, primarily in young men under 35. It is more aggressive than the other form, may or may not respond to treatment, and can spread to other organs. Recently, this type of KS is being seen in organ transplant recipients and cancer patients undergoing chemotherapy.

The KS seen in AIDS patients resembles the African type, primarily striking young homosexual men and aggressively spreading to other organs besides the skin, including the lymph nodes, gastrointestinal organs, and the lungs. The symptoms are painless, nonitching skin lesions, which vary in size from an insect bite to large raised plaques and are colored dark-blue or purple-brown. They may be located anywhere on the skin or mucous membranes, though some patients may have no skin involvement. Often, patients report a history of fevers, night sweats, weight loss, and fatigue.

## WHAT CAUSES AIDS?

Although the proof is not yet absolute, recent evidence points to the human T-cell leukemia virus HTLV-III as the most likely cause, in whole or in part. Its behavior closely parallels the epidemiologic profile of AIDS, that is, it is transmitted by sexual contact, blood transfusion, and intravenous needles, preferentially attacks helper T cells, and can cause malignancies. It has also been isolated in AIDS and AIDS-related complex patients, and antibodies to the virus have been detected in AIDS patients. (The lymphadenopathy virus, or LAV, discovered in France, is thought to be the same as HTLV-III.)

Other candidates that have been considered include herpesviruses such as cytomegalovirus (CMV) and the Epstein-Barr virus (EBV), African swine fever and some other animal viruses endemic to Africa, and even possible mutations of old viruses appearing in a new form. It has also been suggested that immunodeficiency may be the result of a long series of immunologic challenges by common viruses, such as CMV and EBV, that produce an immunodepression which, when aggravated by the presence of other infectious agents, a genetic predisposition, sperm, or toxins, develops into the full-blown clinical disease. A weakness of this multifactorial hypothesis is its failure to satisfactorily explain the appearance of AIDS in infants born to AIDS patients and in some recipients of blood transfusions.

## WHAT ARE THE DIAGNOSTIC TESTS FOR AIDS?

A definitive blood test has yet to be developed. While routine laboratory tests cannot rule out AIDS, they can be useful in indicating the need for more extensive tests of the immune system.

Two routine tests commonly ordered are the white blood cell count and lymphocyte count. Both may be depressed in AIDS patients. Also, healthy people respond to skin tests (injection of special substances called antigens under the top layer of skin) with redness and swelling at the injection site. The absence of such a reaction may indicate that the immune system is not working properly.

When immune deficiency is strongly suspected, the diagnosis may be aided by less routine tests such as lymphocyte subpopulation studies, which measure the number of suppressor and helper lymphocytes in the blood. AIDS patients typically have an abnormally high ratio of suppressor to helper lymphocytes in their blood. They have also been found to have elevated immunoglobulin levels. However, these findings, singly or in combination, are not specific for AIDS. Each is also found in patients with other illnesses.

Blood samples may be taken for special treatment (called blood cultures) to promote the growth of microorganisms. Normally, blood is sterile and should contain no bacteria or other microorganisms. With immune deficiency, however, the body often lacks the defenses to prevent pathogens from multiplying in the blood stream. These foreign organisms constitute an infection, which, with appropriate blood cultures, can be identified and treated.

When a patient belongs to a known risk group for AIDS and has symptoms consistent with opportunistic diseases, the course of action is clear. For suspected Kaposi's sarcoma, a skin sample taken from the affected area is examined microscopically (biopsy) for evidence of Kaposi's sarcoma. Similarly, examination of material obtained from the lung establishes the diagnosis of *Pneumocystis carinii* pneumonia (PCP). Bronchoscopy is an invasive procedure with an illuminated tube inserted down the throat into the airways of the lung, which permits direct inspection of the lung surfaces and sampling tissue for biopsies. If bronchial biopsies do not show PCP and it is still suspected, open-lung biopsy is performed. This involves piercing the skin of the back or chest under anesthesia and obtaining a piece of lung tissue for examination.

## WHAT IS THE T-CELL RATIO AND ITS SIGNIFICANCE?

Lymphocytes are a type of white blood cell involved in the immune response. They can be subdivided into two main groups, B cells and T cells. B-cell lymphocytes are called humoral immunity and are responsible for the manufacture of proteins called immunoglobulins. Immunoglobulins circulate in the blood stream, recognize foreign toxins, and dispose of them. T-cell lymphocytes are called cell-mediated immunity and are effective against intracellular bacteria, viruses, and fungi. T-cell lymphocytes can be further divided into two subclasses, helper T cells and suppressor T cells.

Helper T cells facilitate differentiation and activation of both T and B cells, helping to turn them "on" when needed. We usually have about twice as many helper cells as suppressor cells in our blood. In AIDS, this ratio is reversed, and we have many more suppressor cells than helper cells. The cause of this aberration is not known, but its effect may be lowered resistance against infections such as herpes, yeast, and *Pneumocystis carinii* pneumonia. Its full effect is still not well understood and is under medical investigation.

## HOW DO PERSONS WITH HEMOPHILIA GET AIDS?

Hemophilia is a genetically inherited clotting disorder that affects 15,000–20,000 Americans. An absent or diminished blood-clotting Factor VIII is the cause of abnormal bleeding in some hemophiliacs. Without effective clotting, even minor cuts can cause prolonged, dangerous, and even life-threatening bleeding. For hemophiliacs, the development of Factor VIII concentrate was an important medical advance that vastly improved the quality and span of their lives. Factor VIII is extracted and concentrated from pooled blood plasma donated by thousands of people. Like other blood transfusions, it has the potential for spreading infectious disease. It appears that, in some rare instances, the plasma concentrate may have been contaminated with the putative AIDS agent, and there have been over a dozen cases of AIDS in hemophiliacs who had no other known risk factors for developing the disease.

The Food and Drug Administration has recently instituted a new heat treatment for preparing blood products such as Factor VIII. It is thought that this procedure will reduce the risk of transmitting infections, including AIDS, through blood products.

### CAN AIDS BE CONTRACTED FROM A BLOOD TRANSFUSION?

Possible transfusion-linked AIDS cases have been reported. However, after more than two years of national AIDS surveillance, the observed incidence of AIDS in blood recipients is very low. Statistically, the ratio of the number of units of blood transfused to the few cases of AIDS possibly acquired by transfusion is probably greater than a million to one.

The U.S. Public Health Service has met with blood bank associations and instituted screening procedures to minimize the transfusion risk. In the absence of a specific screening test for AIDS, potential donors are made aware of the general criteria before they come to donate. They are told the facts about AIDS, questioned about present health and past diseases, and advised not to donate blood if they belong to any known risk group or have any symptoms consistent with AIDS. Medical personnel question all donors about fevers, night sweats, unexplained weight loss, a persistent cough, long-lasting diarrhea, bruise-like spots on the skin, and swollen glands. A medical history may be taken and a physical examination given if indicated.

When blood is given, the donor, in private, designates whether the blood is to be used for transfusions or only for research. The donated blood is then labeled with a special code, including the donor's name, removed to a remote station, and processed accordingly.

### IS THERE A DANGER OF CONTRACTING AIDS BY DONATING BLOOD?

Absolutely not. Blood donors do not risk exposure to AIDS. All blood collection centers and blood banks use sterile equipment and disposable needles. AIDS cannot be acquired through blood donation.

## IS THERE ANY RISK OF CONTRACTING AIDS FROM THE NEW HEPATITIS B VACCINE?

There was some concern at first about the safety of the new hepatitis B vaccine. Since it is made from plasma taken from carriers of hepatitis B, and carriers are predominantly homosexual men, a high-risk group for AIDS, many potential vaccine recipients feared that vaccine processing techniques might not inactivate the AIDS agent. However, a review of vaccinated patients has revealed no increased incidence of AIDS.

The vaccine consists of particles of hepatitis virus obtained from the blood of screened, healthy, chronic hepatitis B carriers by a process called plasmapheresis, in which the virus particles are separated from the blood by centrifugation and subjected to a complex sequence of biochemical procedures for the inactivation of viruses. The purification process precludes the survival of any viable viruses, bacteria, or fungal agents, including any likely AIDS agent.

Hepatitis B vaccine is strongly recommended for people, such as homosexual males, intravenous-drug abusers, and certain health-care personnel, at high risk for developing hepatitis.

## SHOULD SPECIAL PRECAUTIONS BE TAKEN BY HOSPITAL PERSONNEL IN THE MANAGEMENT OF AIDS PATIENTS?

Health-care workers appear to have a very low risk of contracting AIDS; almost all reported cases were members of high-risk groups. To date, there has been no evidence of AIDS transmission to hospital personnel from casual contact with AIDS patients or their laboratory specimens. Nonetheless, prudence should be exercised to minimize the risk of transmission of AIDS to hospital employees while still giving AIDS patients optimal care. Precautions should stress avoidance of direct contact of skin and mucous membranes with blood, bodily fluids, secretions, excretions, and tissues from patients judged likely to have AIDS (see table 1 in Chapter 14).

## WHEN SHOULD MASKS BE WORN?

Available epidemiologic data indicate that AIDS is not normally transmitted by the airborne route, so masks are not routinely required. Hospital personnel should wear them only when tending AIDS patients on respirators (mechanical breathing aids) who require frequent suctioning to clear airways, or patients suspected of having tuberculosis or who cough frequently. Visitors entering such patients' rooms should also wear masks. A mask should cover the mouth and nose. A moist mask loses its effectiveness and should be replaced.

### WHEN SHOULD PROTECTIVE EYEWEAR BE WORN?

Protect the eyes wherever blood, bodily fluids, or secretions may be sprayed into the air. For example, a dentist's drill, a cough, or a sneeze can disperse many droplets into the air where they may remain suspended for a long time. Droplets can settle on the surface of the eye and be absorbed into the body.

### WHAT IS THE PURPOSE OF GOWNS?

Gowns prevent the contact of clothes with infective materials. They need not be sterile, but should be disposed of properly. Hands should be washed after the gowns are discarded.

### WHEN SHOULD GLOVES BE WORN?

Gloves are necessary when there is possible contact with an AIDS patient's blood, bodily fluids, or excretions, or with objects or surfaces contaminated by them.

### IS THERE A DANGER OF CONTRACTING AIDS IN GIVING MOUTH-TO-MOUTH RESUSCITATION TO AN AIDS PATIENT?

Although there is evidence that AIDS may be transmitted in blood, it is not clear whether it can be transmitted in saliva. The concern about mouth-to-mouth resuscitation is probably valid because there may be blood in the patient's mouth.

### CAN AIDS PATIENTS USE THE SAME WAITING ROOM AND BATHROOMS AS OTHER PATIENTS?

Yes, according to a report in the *New England Journal of Medicine*, September 22, 1983.

# 17 Health Resources, Hot Lines, and Referral Centers
## VICTOR GONG

The following is a list of organizations and institutions in the major U.S. cities involved in the AIDS crisis. Their number is growing and their character is constantly changing. Some offer counseling, support groups, and crisis intervention, while others give medical evaluations, including diagnostic testing, screening, and patient care; all provide instructive and useful information. These resources are open to everyone, regardless of race, sex, or sexual preference.

Inclusion in this list does not constitute an endorsement of the services rendered. It is intended only as a guide to sources of further information and assistance.

## AIDS ORGANIZATIONS AT THE NATIONAL LEVEL

Gay Rights National Lobby
Box 1892
Washington, DC 20013
(202) 546-1801

KS Research and Education
  Foundation
54 Tenth Street
San Francisco, CA 94103
(415) 864-4376

National Coalition of Gay STD
  Services
P.O. Box 239
Milwaukee, WI 53201
(414) 277-7671

National Gay Task Force
80 Fifth Avenue—Suite 1601
New York, NY 10011
(212) 741-5800
*Crisisline*:
1-800-221-7044
(212) 807-6016 (New York, Alaska,
Hawaii)

Public Health Service
Department of Health and Human
    Services
Washington, DC 20201
(202) 245-6867

## California

### Los Angeles
KS Foundation/Los Angeles
Gay/Lesbian Community Center
1213 North Highland Avenue
Los Angeles, CA 90038
(213) 461-1333

L.A. AIDS Project
937 W. Cole Street—Suite 3
Los Angeles, CA 90038
(213) 871-2437 (Hotline)
(213) 871-1284 (Office)

L.A. Sex Information Hotline
8405 Beverly Boulevard
Los Angeles, CA 90048
(213) 653-2118

Southern California Physicians for
    Human Rights
7985 Santa Monica Boulevard—
    Suite 109
#165
Los Angeles, CA
(213) 658-6261 (Business)
(213) 860-6611

### Sacramento
AIDS & KS Foundation/Sacramento
2115 J Street—Suite #3
Sacramento, CA 95816
(916) 448-AIDS

Beach Area Community Clinic
3705 Mission Blvd.
San Diego, CA 92109
(619) 488-0644

Owen Clinic
University of California
San Diego Medical Center
225 Dickinson Street
San Diego, CA 92103
(619) 294-3995

### San Francisco
American Association of Physi-
    cians for Human Rights
P.O. Box 14366
San Francisco, CA 94114
(415) 673-3189

Bay Area Physicians for Human
    Rights
P.O. Box 14546
San Francisco, CA 94114
(415) 558-9353 (Administration)
(415) 372-7321 (Medical inquiries)

Kaposi's Sarcoma Clinic
University of California, San
    Francisco
Medical Center, A-312
San Francisco, CA 94143
(415) 666-1407

KS Research and Education
    Foundation
54 Tenth Street
San Francisco, CA 94103
(415) 864-4376

Shanti Project
890 Hayes Street
San Francisco, CA 94117
(415) 558-9644

**Colorado**

Colorado AIDS Project
Gay and Lesbian Community Center
1436 Lafayette Street
Denver, CO 80218
(303) 831-6268

Gay and Lesbian Health Alliance
P.O. Box 6101
Denver, CO 80206
(303) 777-9530

**Connecticut**

AIDS Project/New Haven
Box 7
North Haven, CT 06473
(203) 239-7881

Hartford Gay Health Collective
320 Farmington Avenue
Hartford, CT 06105
(203) 527-9813

Yale Self-Care Network
17 Hillhouse Avenue
New Haven, CT 06520

**Delaware**

G.L.A.D.
P.O. Box 9218
Wilmington, DE 19809
1-800-342-4012
(302) 764-2208

**District of Columbia**

Whitman-Walker Clinic
2335 18th Street, NW
Washington, DC 20009
(202) 332-5295

**Florida**

*Miami*

AIDS Support Group
c/o MCC Church
23rd St. & NE 2nd St.
Miami, FL
(305) 573-4156

University of Miami Medical
    School AIDS Project
Department of Medicine R-42
Miami, FL
(305) 325-6338

*Tampa*

University of South Florida
Main Lab, Medical Clinic S.
12901 North 30th Street
Tampa, FL 33612
(813) 974-4214

*Key West*

AIDS Action Committee
Florida Keys Memorial Hospital
P.O. Box 4073
Key West, FL 33041

Monroe County Health Dept.
Public Service Building
Junior College Road
Key West, FL 33040
(305) 294-1021

**Georgia**

AID Atlanta
1801 Piedmont Road
Atlanta, GA 30324
(404) 872-0600

Centers for Disease Control
AIDS Activity
Building 3, Room 5B-1
1600 Clifton Road
Atlanta, GA 30333
(404) 329-3472

**Illinois**

Howard Brown Memorial Clinic
AIDS Action
2676 N. Halstead Street
Chicago, IL 60614
(312) 871-5777 (Office/Medical)
(312) 871-5776 (Hotline)

**Louisiana**

Crescent City Coalition
c/o St. Louis Community Center
1022 Barracks Street
New Orleans, LA 70116
(504) 568-9619

**Maryland**

AIDS Hotline
101 W. Read Street—Suite 815
Baltimore, MD 21201
(301) 244-8484 (Medical Office)
(301) 947-2437

Gay Community Center Clinic
241 W. Chase Street
Baltimore, MD 21201
(301) 837-2050

**Massachusetts**

Boston Department of Health
AIDS Hotline
(617) 424-5916

Fenway Community Health Center,
or AIDS Action Committee
16 Haviland Street
Boston, MA 02215
(617) 267-7573

Mayor's Ad Hoc Committee on
   AIDS
c/o Boston City Hall—Room 608
Boston, MA 02201
(617) 725-4849

**Minnesota**

AIDS Support Group
c/o 2309 Girard Ave. South
Minneapolis, MN 55405

Minnesota AIDS Project
c/o Lesbian & Gay Community
   Services
124 W. Lake St.—Suite E
Minneapolis, MN 55408

**New Hampshire**

New Hampshire Feminist Health
Center
232 Court Street
Portsmouth, NH 03801
(603) 436-6171

**New Jersey**

New Jersey Lesbian and Gay AIDS
Awareness
c/o St. Michaels Medical Center
268 High Street
Newark, NJ 07102
(201) 596-0767

**New York**

Gay Men's Health Crisis
P.O. Box 274
132 W. 24th Street
New York, NY 10011
(212) 685-4952
(212) 807-6655

Gay Men's Health Project
74 Grove Street—#2J
New York, NY 10014
(212) 691-6969

New York City Department of
Health
Office of Gay and Lesbian Health
Concerns
125 Worth Street—#806
New York, NY 10013
(212) 566-6110

St. Mark's Clinic
88 University Place
New York, NY 10003
(212) 691-8282

**Ohio**

*Cincinnati*
Ambrose Clenent Health Clinic
STD Clinic
3101 Burnet Avenue
Cincinnati, OH 45229
(513) 352-3143

*Cleveland*
Cleveland Health Issues
11800 Edgewater Street, #206
Lakewood, OH 44107
(216) 822-7285 (Daytime)
(216) 266-6507 (After 6 pm)

Free Medical Clinic of Greater
Cleveland
12201 Euclid Avenue
Cleveland, OH 44106
(216) 721-4010

**Oklahoma**

Oklahoma Blood Institute
1001 Lincoln Boulevard
Oklahoma City, OK
(405) 239-2437

Oklahomans for Human Rights
1932 "C" South Cheyenne Street
Tulsa, OK 74119
(918) 583-7323

## Oregon

Phoenix Rising/Cascade AIDS
  Project
408 Southwest 2nd Ave.—Room
  403
Portland, OR 97204
(503) 223-8299

## Pennsylvania

### Philadelphia

AIDS Task Force
c/o Philadelphia City Health
  Department
P.O. Box 7529
Philadelphia, PA 19101
(215) 574-9666 (Office)
(215) 232-8055 (Hotline)

Philadelphia Community Health
  Alternatives
P.O. Box 7259
Philadelphia, PA 19109
(215) 624-2879

### Pittsburgh

Graduate School of Public Health
University of Pittsburgh Health
  Center
A-417 Crabtree Hall
Pittsburgh, PA 15261
(412) 624-3928
(412) 624-3331

## Texas

### Dallas

AIDS Action Project
c/o Oaklawn Counseling Center
Suite 202
3409 Oaklawn Street
Dallas, TX 75219
(214) 528-2181

### Houston

KS/AIDS Foundation of Houston
3317 Montrose Boulevard
Houston, TX 77006
(713) 524-2437

The Montrose Clinic
104 Westheimer
Houston, TX 77006
(713) 528-5531
(713) 528-5535

### San Antonio

Safeweek/AIDS Committee
1713 West Mulberry
San Antonio, TX 78201
(512) 736-5216

## Washington

Gay Men's Health Group
2353 Minor Ave. E.
Seattle, WA 98102
(206) 322-3919

Harbor View Medical Center
STD Clinic
324 9th—ZA-85
Seattle, WA 98104
(206) 223-3000

NW AIDS Foundation
P.O. Box 3449
Seattle, WA 98114
(206) 527-8770
(206) 622-9650


**Wisconsin**

*Madison*

Blue Bus Clinic
1552 University Avenue
Madison, WI 53706
(608) 262-7440

*Milwaukee*

Brady East STD Clinic
1240 East Brady Street
Milwaukee, WI 53202
(414) 272-2144

National Coalition of Gay Sexually
Transmitted Disease Services
(NCGSTDS)
P.O. Box 239
Milwaukee, WI 53201

# Glossary

**Acyclovir**: A new antiviral agent

**AIDS**: Acquired immune deficiency syndrome

**Aids-related complex (ARC)**: A heterogeneous group of clinical disorders in high-risk individuals, related to but not necessarily prodromal for AIDS, including diffuse lymphadenopathy, fever, profound fatigue, weight loss, and diarrhea. ARC is usually accompanied by depressed cell-mediated immunity similar to but less severe than that found in AIDS.

**Anemia**: A condition in which the number of red blood cells is reduced

**Antibody**: A protein made by the immune system to inactivate antigens and help fight infections

**Antigen**: A foreign substance that activates the immune system

**Autoimmune disease**: A condition in which the body's immune system attacks its own tissues

**Antibiotic**: A drug used to fight bacterial infection

**Bacterium**: A one-celled microscopic organism

**Biopsy**: Removal of a tissue sample for examination to establish a diagnosis

**Blood count**: A laboratory test to determine the number of red cells, white cells, and platelets in the blood

**Bone marrow**: A soft material in the center of bones where blood cells are manufactured

**Bone marrow transplant**: Removal of bone marrow from a donor and transfusion of the marrow into a recipient

**Cancer**: A group of diseases characterized by an uncontrolled growth of abnormal cells that can destroy surrounding tissues and spread to other organs of the body

**Candidiasis**: A yeast infection that typically affects the tongue, mouth, and esophagus (oral thrush), appearing as white, curdlike patches

**Chemotherapy**: Administration of anticancer drugs

**Cryptosporidiosis**: An infection due to a protozoan, commonly seen in cattle and cattle handlers, that usually causes a self-limiting diarrhea but, in AIDS, results in severe diarrhea that can lead to dehydration and malnutrition

**Cytomegalovirus**: A virus of the herpes family that can cause illnesses that range from flu-like infections to hepatitis, pneumonia, and brain infections

**Encephalitis**: A serious infection of brain tissue

**Endemic**: Present in the community at all times (usually referring to a disease)

**Epidemic**: A disease that affects many people in a particular area at the same time

**Epidemiology**: The study of the relationships of various factors to the incidence and distribution of a disease

**Etiology**: The cause(s) or origin(s) of diseases

**Fungus**: A member of the plant family that includes yeast, molds, mildew, and mushrooms

**Gastrointestinal**: Pertaining to organs of the digestive system

**Hemophilia**: A hereditary blood-clotting disorder that almost exclusively affects males

**Hepatitis**: Inflammation of the liver, causing jaundice, vomiting, malaise, fevers, and abdominal pain

**Iatrogenic**: Resulting from the activities of a physician

**Incidence**: Number of cases of a disease occurring during a given period

**Incubation period**: The lapse of time from the entry of a germ into the body to the appearance of disease symptoms

**Intravenous**: Into the vein

**Immunity**: The body's ability to resist disease by a system of defense mechanisms, including the action of antibodies, various white blood cells, and other agents

**Immunotherapy**: A treatment of cancer and other diseases with substances that enhance the body's own natural defenses

**Immunodeficient**: Having an impaired or nonfunctioning immune system

**Immunomodulation**: Attempts to change the body's immune responses (e.g., to restore an AIDS-impaired immune system back to normal)

**Interferon/Interleukin**: White blood cell products, called lymphokines, found at abnormal levels in AIDS patients. Interferon is a protein made by the lymphocyte that prevents viruses from infecting other cells.

**Lymphocytes**: White blood cells, called B cells (bursa-dependent) or T cells (thymus-dependent), that are an important part of the immune system

**Lymph nodes**: Glands that fight infection by filtering out germs and producing antibodies, and that usually become swollen when infection, cancer, drug reactions, or other disease conditions exist in the body

**Lymphatic system**: A circulatory system of vessels, spaces, and lymph nodes that fights infection

**Lymphomas**: Cancers of the lymphatic system

**Malignant**: Cancerous

**Meningitis**: A serious infection of the membranes surrounding the brain

**Metastasis**: Spread of cancer from one part of the body to another to form new tumors

**Morbidity**: Condition of being diseased

**Natural killer cells**: T cells important in the body's destruction of tumor cells

**Neoplasm**: An abnormal growth of tissue, either benign or malignant

**Opportunistic infection**: Infection by a microorganism that may be common in the environment but causes disease only in a host with a poorly functioning immune system

**Parasite**: An organism that depends on food from a host for survival

**Plasmapheresis**: A sophisticated form of filtration that separates cells and other products from blood

**Platelet**: A component of blood that helps in clotting and wound healing

**Prevalence:** Number of cases of a disease existing at a given time

**Prodrome**: A collection of signs and symptoms that may precede the onset of overt disease

**Protozoa**: One-celled microscopic animals

**Radiation therapy**: Treatment of cancer with high-energy radiation such as x-rays

**Red blood cells**: Disc-shaped blood components that carry oxygen to body tissues

**Reticuloendothelial system**: A part of the immune system involved with phagocytosis (engulfing and destroying) of antigens

**T-cell helper/suppressor ratio**: Ratio of number of helper T cells to number of suppressor T cells, normally 2 to 1 in a healthy person, but reversed in AIDS

**Thymus**: A gland in the neck intimately connected with T-cell properties

**Tumor**: A swelling or neoplasm that may be cancerous

**Virus**: A microscopic noncellular organism that depends on a living host cell for survival and causes many common diseases such as the common cold, measles, mumps, and chicken pox

**White blood cells**: Blood cells that fight infection

# References and Sources

## Chapter 1. AIDS—Defining the Syndrome

Centers for Disease Control: Persistent generalized lymphadenopathy among homosexual males. *Morb Mortal Wkly Rep* 1982; 31:249–251

————. Acquired immunodeficiency syndrome update. *Morb Mortal Wkly Rep* 1983; 32:465–467

————. Update: Acquired immunodeficiency syndrome (AIDS)—United States. *Morb Mortal Wkly Rep* 1984; 32:688–691

Fauci A et al. Acquired immunodeficiency syndrome: Epidemiologic, clinical, immunologic, and therapeutic considerations. *Ann Intern Med* 1984; 100:92–106

Friedman-Kien AE, Laubstein LJ, Rubinstein P, Buimovici-Kien E, et al. Disseminated Kaposi's sarcoma in homosexual men. *Ann Intern Med* 1982; 96 (Part 1):693–700

Gong V. Acquired immunodeficiency syndrome. *Am J Emergency Room Med* 1984; 2(4):336–346

Haverkos HW and Curran JW: The current outbreaks of Kaposi's sarcoma and opportunistic infections. *Cancer J Clin* 1982; 32(6)

Masur H. The acquired immunodeficiency syndrome. *DM* 1983; 30(1):5–48

Masur H, Michelis MA, Grene JB, et al. An outbreak of community-acquired *Pneumocystis carinii* pneumonia: initial manifestations of a cellular immune dysfunction. *N Eng J Med* 1981; 305:1431–1438

Morris L, Distenfeld A, Amorosi E, and Karpatkin S. Autoimmune thrombocytopenia purpura in homosexual men. *Ann Intern Med* 1982; 96:705–713

Scott GB, Buck BE, Letterman JG, Bloom FL, and Parks WP. Acquired immunodeficiency syndrome in infants. *N Engl J Med* 1984; 310:76–81

**Chapter 2.    Assembling the AIDS Puzzle: Epidemiology**

Centers for Disease Control. Pneumocystis Pneumonia—Los Angeles. *Morb Mortal Wkly Rep* 1981; 30:250–252

――――. Kaposi's sarcoma and Pneumocystis pneumonia among homosexual men—New York City and California. *Morb Mortal Wkly Rep* 1981; 30: 305–308

――――. *Pneumocystis carinii* pneumonia and mucosal candidiasis in previously healthy homosexual men. Evidence of a new acquired cellular immunodeficiency. *N Engl J Med* 1981; 305:1425–1431

――――. Persistent, generalized lymphadenopathy among homosexual males. *Morb Mortal Wkly Rep* 1981; 30:249–251

――――. Diffuse, undifferentiated non-Hodgkin's lymphoma among homosexual males—United States. *Morb Mortal Wkly Rep* 1982; 31:277– 279

――――. Update on Kaposi's sarcoma and opportunistic infections in previously healthy persons—United States. *Morb Mortal Wkly Rep* 1982; 31:291–301

――――. Update on Kaposi's sarcoma among Haitians in the United States. *Morb Mortal Wkly Rep* 1982; 31:353–361

――――. A cluster of Kaposi's sarcoma and *Pneumocystis carinii* pneumonia among homosexual male residents of Los Angeles and Orange counties, California. *Morb Mortal Wkly Rep* 1982; 31:305–307

――――. *Pneumocystis carinii* pneumonia among persons with hemophilia A. *Morb Mortal Wkly Rep* 1982; 31:355–357

――――. Update on acquired immune deficiency syndrome (AIDS) among patients with hemophilia A. *Morb Mortal Wkly Rep* 1982; 31:644–652

――――. Possible transfusion-associated acquired immune deficiency syndrome (AIDS)—California. *Morb Mortal Weekly Rep* 1982; 31:652–654

Centers for Disease Control Task Force. Special Report: Epidemiologic aspects of the current outbreak of Kaposi's sarcoma and opportunistic infections. *N Engl J Med* 1982; 306:248–252

Clumeck N, Sennet S, Taelman H, et al. Acquired immunodeficiency syndrome in African patients. *N Engl J Med* 1984; 310(8):492–497

Gottlieb MS, Schroff R, Schanker HM, et al. *Pneumocystis carinii* pneumonia and mucosal candidiasis in previously healthy homosexual men; evidence of a new acquired cellular immunodeficiency. *N Engl J Med* 1981; 305:1425–1431

Groopman JE and Volberding PA. The AIDS epidemic: Continental drift. *Nature* 1984; 307(19):211–212

Marx JL. Acquired immune deficiency syndrome abroad. *Science* 1983; 222:998–999

## Chapter 3.    The Immunology of AIDS

Ammann AJ, Abrams D, Conant M, et al. Acquired immune dysfunction in homosexual men: Immunological profiles. *Clin Immunol and Immunopath* 1983; 27:315–325

Hokama Y and Nakamura RM. *Immunology and Immunopathology. Basic Concepts.* Little, Brown, Boston, 1982

Reuben JM, Hersh EM, Mansell P, et al. Immunological characterization of homosexual males. *Cancer Research* 1983; 43:897–904

Rogers MF, Morens DM, Stewart JA, et al., and the Task Force on Acquired Immune Deficiency Syndrome. National case-control study of Kaposi's sarcoma and *Pneumocystis carinii* pneumonia in homosexual men: Part 2, Laboratory Results. *Ann Intern Med* 1983; 99:151–158

Rose NR, Migrom F, and van Oss C. *Principles of Immunology*, Second Edition. MacMillan, New York, 1979

Rubinstein A, Sicklick M, Gupta A, et al. Acquired immunodeficiency with reversed $T_4/T_8$ ratios in infants born to promiscuous and drug-addicted mothers. *J Am Med Assoc* 1983; 249:2350–2356

Small CB, Klein RS, Friedland GH, et al. Community-acquired opportunistic infections and defective cellular immunity in heterosexual drug abusers and homosexual men. *Am J Med* 1983; 74:433–441

Stahl RE, Friedman-Kien AE, Dubin R, et al. Immunologic abnormalities in homosexual men. Relationship to Kaposi's sarcoma. *Am J Med* 1982; 73:171–178

## Chapter 4.    Signs and Symptoms of AIDS

Britton CB, Marquardt MD, Koppel B, Garvey G, and Miller JR. Neurological complications of the gay immunosuppressed syndrome: Clinical and pathological features. (Abstract). *Ann Neurology* 1982; 12(1):80

Buimovici-Kiein E et al. Disseminated Kaposi's sarcoma in homosexual men. *Ann Intern Med* 1982; 96 (Part 1):693–700

Centers for Disease Control. Acquired immune deficiency syndrome (AIDS): Precautions for clinical and laboratory staffs. *Morb Mortal Wkly Rep* 1982; 31(43):577–580

———. An evaluation of the acquired immunodeficiency syndrome (AIDS) reported in health-care personnel—United States. *Morb Mortal Wkly Rep* 1983; 32(27):358–360

———. Cryptosporidiosis: Assessment of chemotherapy of males with acquired immunodeficiency syndrome. *Morb Mortal Wkly Rep* 1982; 31:589–592

Centers for Disease Control Task Force on Kaposi's Sarcoma and Opportunistic Infections. Epidemiological aspects of the current outbreak of Kaposi's sarcoma and opportunistic infections. *N Engl J Med* 1982; 306: 248–252

Follansbee SE, Busch DF, Wofsy CB, et al. An outbreak of *Pneumocystis carinii* pneumonia in homosexual men. *Ann Intern Med* 1982; 96:539–546

Friedman-Kien AE, Laubenstein L, Marmor M, et al. Kaposi's sarcoma and pneumocystis pneumonia among homosexual men—New York and California. *Morb Mortal Wkly Rep* 1981; 30:305–308

Gopinathan G, Laubenstein LJ, Mondale B, and Krigel RL. Central nervous system manifestations of the acquired immune deficiency syndrome in homosexual men. (Abstract), *Neurology* 1983; 33 (Suppl 2):105

Gottlieb MS, Schroff R, Schanker HM, et al. *Pneumocystis carinii* pneumonia and mucosal candidiasis in previously healthy homosexual men: Evidence of a new acquired cellular immunodeficiency. *N Engl J Med* 1981; 305:1425–1431

Greene JB, Sidu GS, Leein S, et al. *Mycobacterium avium-intracellulare*. A cause of disseminated life-threatening infection in homosexuals and drug abusers. *Ann Intern Med* 1982; 97:539–546

Herman P. Neurologic complications of acquired immunologic deficiency syndrome. (Abstract). *Neurology* 1983; 33 (Suppl 2):105

Masur H, Michelis MA, Grene JB, et al. An outbreak of community-acquired *Pneumocystis carinii* pneumonia: Initial manifestations of a cellular immune dysfunction. *N Engl J Med* 1981; 305:1431–1438

Mildvan D, Mathur U, Enlow R, et al. Opportunistic infections and immune deficiency in homosexual men. *Ann Intern Med* 1982; 96 (Part I):700–704

Miller JR, Barrett RE, Britton CB, et al. Progressive multifocal leukoencephalopathy in a male with T-cell immune deficiency. *N Engl J Med* 1983; 307:1436–1437

Morris L, Distendfeld A, Amorosi E, and Karpatkin S. Autoimmune thrombocytopenic purpura in homosexual men. *Ann Intern Med* 1982; 96:714–717

Pitchenik AE, Fischi MA, Dickinson GM, et al. Opportunistic infections and Kaposi's sarcoma among Haitians: Evidence of a new acquired immunodeficiency state. *Ann Intern Med* 1983; 98:277–284

Post MH, Chan JC, Hensley GT, Hoffman TA, Moskowitz LB, and Lippman S. Toxoplasma encephalitis in Haitian adults with acquired immunodeficiency syndrome: A clinical-pathologic CT correlation. *Am J Roentgenology* 1983; 140:861–868

Snider WD, Simpson DM, Aronyk KE, and Nielson SL. Primary lymphoma of the nervous system associated with acquired immune deficiency syndrome. *N Engl J Med* 1983; 308:45

Snider WD, Simpson DM, Nielsen S, et al. Neurological complications of acquired immune deficiency syndrome: Analysis of 50 patients. *Ann Neurology* 1983; 14(4):403–418

## Chapter 5.    The Infections of AIDS

### 5A.  *Viral Infections*

Barre-Senoussi F, Chermann JC, Rey F, et al. Isolation of a T-lymphocyte retrovirus from a patient at risk of acquired immunodeficiency syndrome. *Science* 1983; 220:868–870

Cawson RA, McCracken AW, and Marcus PB. *Pathologic Mechanisms and Human Disease*. C V Mosby, St. Louis, 1982

Essex M, McLane MF, and Lee TH: Antibodies to cell membrane antigens associated with human T-cell leukemia virus in patients with A.I.D.S. *Science* 1983; 220:859–862

Gallo RC. The Virus-cancer story. *Hospital Practice*, June 1983

Gallo RC, Sarin PS, and Gelman EP. Isolation of human T-cell leukemia virus in acquired immune deficiency syndrome. *Science* 1983; 220:865–867

Gelman EP, Popovic M, Blayney D, Masur H, et al. Proviral DNA of a retrovirus, human T-cell leukemia virus in patients with A.I.D.S. *Science* 1983; 220:862–865

Lennette EH and Schmidt NJ. *Diagnostic Procedures for Viral, Rickettsial and Chlamydial Infections*, Fifth Edition. American Public Health Association, Washington, DC, 1979

Lipscomb H, Tatsumi E, Harada S, et al. Epstein-Barr virus and chronic lymphadenomegaly in male homosexuals with acquired immunodeficiency syndrome (AIDS). *AIDS Research* 1983; 1(1), 59–82

Peter JB and Wolde-Mariam W. AIDS: Putting the pieces together. *Diagn Med*, Feb 1984, pp 56–65

Sonnabend J, Witkin SS, and Purtilo DT. Acquired immunodeficiency syndrome, opportunistic infections and malignancies in male homosexuals. *J Am Med Assoc* 1983; 249, 2370–2374

### 5B.   *Parasitic Infections*

Baker RW and Peppercorn MA. Enteric disease of homosexual men. *Pharmacotherapy* 1982; 2(1):21–32

―――. Gastrointestinal ailments of homosexual men. *Medicine* 1982; 61(6):390–405

Centers for Disease Control. Cryptosporidiosis: Assessment of chemotherapy of males with acquired immune deficiency syndrome (AIDS). *Morb Mortal Wkly Rep* 1982; 31:589–592

Centers for Disease Control Task Force on Kaposi's sarcoma and opportunistic infections. Epidemiologic aspects of the current outbreak of Kaposi's sarcoma and opportunistic infections. *N Engl J Med* 1982; 306: 248–252

Chandra RK. Immune responses in parasitic diseases. Part B: Mechanisms. *Rev Infect Dis* 1983; 4(4):756

Cruickshank JK and Mackensie C. Immunodiagnosis in parasitic disease. *Brit Med J* 1981; 283:1349–1350

Hakes T and Armstrong D. Toxoplasmosis: Problems in diagnosis and treatment. *Cancer* 1983; 20:1535–1540

Huges WT, Feldman S, et al. Comparison of pentamidine isethionate and trimethoprim-sulfamethoxazole in the treatment of *Pneumocystis carinii* pneumonia. *J Pediatr* 1978; 92:285–291

Kean BH. Clinical amebiasis in New York City: Symptoms, signs and treatment. *Bull NY Acad Med* 1981; 57:207

Keusch GT. Immune responses in parasitic diseases. Part A. General concepts. *Rev Infect Dis* 1983; 4(4):751–755

Krogstad DJ, Spencer HC Jr, and Healy GR. Current concepts in parasitology: Amebiasis. *N Engl J Med* 1978; 298:262–265

Landesman SH and Viera J. Acquired immune deficiency syndrome (AIDS)—A review. *Arch Intern Med* 1983; 143:2307–2309

Salfelder K and Schwarz V. Pneumocystosis. *Am J Dis Child* 1967; 114:693–699

Smith JW and Wolfe MS. Giardiasis. *Ann Rev Med* 1980; 31:373–383

Tzipori S. Cryptosporidiosis in animals and humans. *Microbiol Rev* 1983; 47:84–96

Walzer PD, Perl DP, et al. *Pneumocystis carinii* pneumonia in the United States. Epidemiologic, diagnostic and clinical features. *Ann Intern Med* 1974: 80:83–93

Wong B. Parasitic diseases in immunocompromised hosts. *Am J Med* 1983; 76:479–485.

### 5C.   Bacterial and Fungal Infections

Centers for Disease Control Task Force on Kaposi's sarcoma and opportunistic infections. Epidemiological aspects of the current outbreak of Kaposi's sarcoma and opportunistic infections. *N Engl J Med* 1982; 306:248–252

Dutt AK and Stead W. Long-term results of medical treatment in *Mycobacterium intracellulare* infection. *Am J Med* 1979; 67:449–453

Greene JB, Sidhu GS, Lewin S, et al. *Mycobacterium avium-intracellulare*: A cause of disseminated life-threatening infection in homosexuals and drug abusers. *Ann Intern Med* 1982; 97(4):539–546

Gottlieb M et al. The acquired immunodeficiency syndrome—UCLA conference. *Ann Intern Med* 1983; 99:208–220

Kaufman CA, Israel KS, Smith JW, et al. Histoplasmosis in immunosuppressed patients. *Am J Med* 1978; 64:923

Krick JR and Remington JS. Resistance to infection with *Nocardia asteroides*. *J Infect Dis* 1975; 142:432

Lane HC, Masur H, Edgar LC, et al. Abnormalities of B-cell activation and immunoregulation in patients with the acquired immunodeficiency syndrome. *N Engl J Med* 1983; 309(8):453–458

Louria DB. Bacterial and fungal infections in AIDS. In *The AIDS Epidemic*, ed. K Cahill. St. Martin's, New York, 1983

Mildvan D, Mathur U, Enlow R, et al. Opportunistic infections and immune deficiency in homosexual men. *Ann Intern Med* 1982; 96 (Part I):700–704

Pitchenik AE, Fischi MA, Dickinson GM, et al. Opportunistic infections and Kaposi's sarcoma among Haitians: Evidence of a new acquired immunodeficiency state. *Ann Intern Med* 1983; 98:277–284

Rosenzweig D. Pulmonary mycobacterial infections due to *Mycobacterium intracellulare-avium* complex. *Chest* 1979; 75(2):115–119

Wolinsky E. Nontuberculous mycobacteria and associated disease *Am Rev Resp Dis* 1979; 119:107–159

Yeager H and Raleigh J. Pulmonary diseases due to *Mycobacterium intracellulare. Am Rev Resp Dis* 1973; 108:547–552

Zakowiski P, Fligiel S, et al. Disseminated *Mycobacterium avium-intracellulare* infection in homosexual men dying of acquired immunodeficiency. *J Am Med Assoc* 1982; 248(22):2980–2982

## Chapter 6.    Cancers and AIDS

Ammann AJ, Ashman RF, Buckley RH, et al. Use of intravenous gamma globulin in antibody immunodeficiency: Results of a multicenter controlled trial. *Clin Immunol and Immunopath* 1982; 22:60–67

Bartal AH, Lichtig CH, Friedmann-Birnbaum R, et al. The study of classical Kaposi's sarcoma with mouse monoclonal antibodies to human sarcoma and connective tissue differentiation antigen. *Proceedings Am Soc Clin Oncol* 1984; Vol 3 (March 1984): 15 (Abstr C-58)

Biggar RJ, Winn DM, Grossman RJ, et al. Determinant of lesser AIDS. *Proceedings Am Soc Clin Oncol* 1984; Vol 3 (March 1984): 14 (Abstr C-55)

Bussel JB, Kimberly RP, Inman RD, et al. Intravenous gamma globulin for chronic idiopathic thrombocytopenic purpura. *Blood* 1983; 62(2):480–486

Chaganti RSK, Jhanwar SC, Koziner B, et al. Specific translocations characterize Burkitt's-like lymphoma of homosexual men with the acquired immunodeficiency syndrome. *Blood* 1983; 61:1269–1272

Cioanu N, Andreef M, Safai B, et al. Lymphoblastic neoplasia in a homosexual patient with Kaposi's sarcoma. *Ann Intern Med* 1983; 98:151–155

Conant MA, Volberding P, Fletcher V, et al. Squamous cell carcinoma in sexual partners of Kaposi's sarcoma patient. *Lancet* 1982; i:286

Cooper HS, Patchefsky AS, and Marks G. Cloacogenic carcinoma of the anorectum in homosexual men: An observation of four cases. *Dis Col and Rect* 1979; 557–558

DiGiovanna JJ and Safai B. Kaposi's sarcoma. Retrospective study of 90 cases with particular emphasis on the familial occurrence, ethnic background and prevalence of other diseases. *Am J Med* 1981; 71:779–783

Doll DC and List AF. Burkitt's lymphoma in a homosexual. *Lancet* 1982; i:1026–1027

Fehr J, Hofmann V, and Kappeler V. Transient reversal of thrombocytopenic purpura by high-dose intravenous gamma globulin. *N Engl J Med* 1982; 306:1254.

Friedman-Kien AE, Lauberstein LJ, Rubinstein P, et al. Disseminated Kaposi's sarcoma in homosexual men. *Am J Med* 1982; 96 (Part I): 693–700

Gallo RC, Salahuddin SZ, and Popovic M. Frequent detection and isolation of cytopathic retroviruses (HTLV-III) from patients with AIDS and at risk for AIDS. *Science* 1984; 224 (4648):500–503

Gerstoft J, Malchow-Miller A, Bygbjerg I, et al. Severe acquired immunodeficiency in European homosexual men. *Brit Med J* 1982; 285:17–19

Haverkos HW and Curran JW. The current outbreak of Kaposi's sarcoma and opportunistic infection. *CA* 1982; 32:330–339

Kaposi M. Idiopathisches multiples pigmentsarkom der. *Haut Arch Der matol Syph* 1972; 4:265–273

Kondlaponoodi P. Anorectal cancer and homosexuality. *J Am Med Assoc* 1982; 248:2114–2115

Krown SE, Real FX, Cunningham-Rundles S, et al. Preliminary observations on the effects of recombinant leukocyte A interferon in homosexual men with Kaposi's sarcoma. *N Engl J Med* 1983; 308:1071–1076

Lauberstein L, Hymes K, Krigel R. Phase II trial of VP-16213 in disseminated Kaposi's sarcoma. *Proceedings Am Soc Clin Oncol* 1982; (C-680): 174

Leach RD and Ellis H. Carcinoma of the rectum in male homosexuals. *J Roy Soc Med* 1981; 74:490–491

Levine AS. The epidemic of acquired immune dysfunction in homosexual men and its sequelae—opportunistic infections, Kaposi's sarcoma and other malignancies: An update and interpretation. *Cancer Treat Rep* 1982; 66:1391–1395

Mitsuyasu RT and Groopman JE. Biology and therapy of Kaposi's sarcoma. *Seminars Oncology* 1984; Vol 11 (No. 1 March): 53–59

Morris L, Distenfeld A, and Amorosi E. Autoimmune thrombocytopenic pupura in homosexual men. *Ann Intern Med* 1982; 96:714–717

Nydegger VE, ed. *Immunochemotherapy: A Guide to Immunoglobulin Prophylaxia and Therapy.* Academic Press, New York, 1981

Poiesz B, Tomar R, Ehrlich G, et al. Association of HTLV with AIDS. *Proceedings Am Soc Clin Oncol* 1984; Vol 3 (March 1984): 13 (Abstr C-52)

Rosen FS, Cooper MD, and Wedgwood RJP. The primary immunodeficiency. *N Engl J Med* 1984; 311:235-242

Safai B and Good RA. Kaposi's sarcoma: A review and recent developments. *CA* 1981; 31:2-12

Schoeppel SL, Hoppe RT, Dorfman RF, et al. Hodgkin's disease in homosexual men at risk for AIDS. *Proceedings Am Soc Clin Oncol* 1984; Vol 3 (March 1984): 64 (Abstr C-250)

Tosi P, Avteri A, and Cintovino M. Angioimmunoblastic lymphadenopathy with dysproteinemia complicated by Kaposi's sarcoma. *Tumor* 1979; 65: 363-371

Volberding P. Therapy of Kaposi's sarcoma in AIDS. *Seminars Oncology* 1984; Vol 11 (No. 1 March): 60-67

Weldon-Linne CM, Rhone DP, Blatt D, et al. Angiolipomas in homosexual men. *N Engl J Med* 1984; 310:1192-1194

## Chapter 7.    The Elusive Etiology—Possible Causes and Pathogenesis of AIDS

Aledort LM. AIDS: An update. *Hospital Practice* September 1983

Barre-Senoussi F, Chermann JC, Rey F, et al. Isolation of a T-lymphotropic retrovirus from a patient at risk of acquired immunodeficiency syndrome. *Science* 1983; 220:868-871

Curran JW. AIDS—Two years later. Editorial, *N Engl J Med* 1983; 309: 609-611

Goedert JJ et al. Amyl nitrite may alter T-lymphocytes in homosexual men. *Lancet* 1982; i:215-412

Levy JA and Ziegler JL. Acquired immunodeficiency syndrome is an opportunistic infection and Kaposi's sarcoma results from secondary immune stimulation. *Lancet* 1983; ii:78-91

London WT et al. Experimental transmission of simian acquired immunodeficiency syndrome and Kaposi-like skin lesions. *Lancet* 1983; ii:869-873

Popovic M, Sarngadharan MG, Read E, et al. Detection, isolation, and continuous production of cytopathic retroviruses (HTLV-3) from patients with AIDS and pre-AIDS. *Science* 1984; 224:497-500

Shearer GM and Hurtenbach U. Is sperm immunosuppressive in male homosexuals and vasectomized men? *Immunology Today* 1982; 3:153-154

Sonnabend J, Witkin SS, and Purtilo DT. Acquired immunodeficiency syndrome, opportunistic infections and malignancies in male homosexuals. *J Am Med Assoc* 1983; 249:2370-2374

### Chapter 8.    The Haitian Link

Centers for Disease Control. Update on acquired immune deficiency syndrome (AIDS)—United States. *Morb Mortal Wkly Rep* 1982; 31:507–508

Frank E, Siegal FP, Siegal M, Vieira J, et al. T-cell subsets in Haitians with tuberculosis (TB): Predictive value for acquired immune deficiency syndrome (AIDS). (Abstract) *23rd Interscience Conference on Antimicrobial Agents and Chemotherapy* 1983; 261

Harwood A, ed. *Ethnicity and Medical Care: Haitian Americans.* Harvard University Press, Cambridge, 1979

Leonides JR and Hyppolite N. Haiti and the acquired immunodeficiency syndrome. *Ann Intern Med* 1983; 98:1020–1021

Lundahl M. *Peasants and Poverty: A Study in Haiti.* Croom Helm, London, 1979

Macek C. Acquired immunodeficiency syndrome cause(s) still elusive. *J Am Med Assoc* 1982; 248:1423–1431

Metraux A. *La Voudou Haitien.* Gallimard, Paris, 1958; 150–157

Pape JW, Liautaud B, Thomas F, Mathurin JR, et al. Characteristics of the acquired immunodeficiency syndrome (AIDS) in Haiti. *N Engl J Med* 1983; 309:945–950

Pearce RB. Intestinal protozoal infections and AIDS (letter). *Lancet* 1983; 2:51

Pitchenik AE, Fischl MA, Dickenson GM, Becker DM, et al. Opportunistic infections and Kaposi's sarcoma among Haitians: Evidence of a new acquired immunodeficiency state. *Ann Intern Med* 1983; 98:277–284

Vieira J, Frank E, Spira TJ, and Landesman SH. Acquired immune deficiency in Haitians: Opportunistic infections in previously healthy Haitian immigrants. *N Engl J Med* 1983; 308:125–129


### Chapter 9.    Hemophiliacs, Blood Transfusions, and AIDS

Aach RD et al. Serum alanine aminotransferase of donors in relation to the risk of non-A, non-B hepatitis in recipients. *N Engl J Med* 1981; 304:989

Centers for Disease Control. Possible transfusion-associated acquired immunodeficiency syndrome (AIDS)—California. *Morb Mortal Wkly Rep* 1982; 31:652

———. The safety of hepatitis B virus vaccine. *Morb Mortal Wkly Rep* 1983; 32:134

———. Transfusion malaria. *Morb Mortal Wkly Rep* 1983; 32:222

———. Update: Acquired immunodeficiency syndrome (AIDS) among patients with hemophilia A. *Morb Mortal Wkly Rep* 1983; 32:613

————. Update: Acquired immunodeficiency syndrome (AIDS)—United States. *Morb Mortal Wkly Rep* 1984; 32:688

Curran JW et al. Acquired immunodeficiency syndrome (AIDS) associated with transfusion. *N Engl J Med* 1984; 310:69

Feorino PM, Kalyanaraman VS, Haverkos HW, et al. Lymphadenopathy associated virus infection of a blood donor-recipient pair with acquired immunodeficiency syndrome. *Science* 1984; 225:69

Gallo RC et al. Frequent detection and isolation of cytopathic retrovirus (HTLV-III) from patients with AIDS and at risk for AIDS. *Science* 1984; 224:500

Klatzmann D et al. Selective tropism of lymphadenopathy associated virus (LAV) for helper-inducer T lymphocytes. *Science* 1984; 225:59

*Recommendations to Decrease the Risk of Transmitting Infectious Diseases from Blood Donors.* Office of Biologics, National Center for Drugs and Biologics, Food and Drug Administration, Bethesda, MD, March 1983

Stevens C. Correspondence. *N Engl J Med* 1983; 308:1163

**Chapter 10.   Is the General Public at Risk?**

Ammann AJ. Is there an acquired immune deficiency syndrome in infants and children? *Pediatrics* 1983; 72:430

Centers for Disease Control. An evaluation of the acquired immunodeficiency syndrome (AIDS) reported in Health-Care Personnel—United States. *Morb Mortal Wkly Rep* 1983; 32:358

Curran JW. AIDS—Two years later. *N Engl J Med* 1983; 309:609

Feorino PM, Kalyanaraman VS, Haverkos HW, et al. Lymphadenopathy associated virus infection of a blood donor recipient pair with acquired immunodeficiency syndrome. *Science* 1984, 225:69

Gordon RS. *AIDS Memorandum* 1983; 1:11

Groopman JE et al. HTLV-III in saliva of people with AIDS-related complex and healthy homosexual men at risk for AIDS. *Science* 1984; 226:449

Harris C, Butkus-Small C, Klein RS, et al. Immunodeficiency in female sexual partners of men with the acquired immunodeficiency syndrome. *N Engl J Med* 1983; 308:1181

Ho DD et al. HTLV-III in the semen and blood of a healthy homosexual man. *Science* 1984; 226:451

Oleske J, Minneror A, Cooper, R Jr, et al. Immunodeficiency syndrome in children. *J Am Med Assoc* 1983; 249:2345

Popovic M, Sarngadharan MG, Read E, and Gallo RC. Detection, isolation, and continuous production of cytopathic retroviruses (HTLV-111) from patients with AIDS and pre-AIDS. *Science* 1984; 224:497

Rubinstein A. Editorial: Acquired immunodeficiency syndrome in infants. *Am J Dis Child* 1983; 137:825

Rubinstein A, Sicklick M, Gupta A, et al. Acquired immunodeficiency with reversed $T_4/T_8$ ratios in infants born to promiscuous and drug addicted mothers. *J Am Med Assoc* 1983; 249:2350

### Chapter 11.  Ethical Issues in AIDS

Bayer R, Levine C, and Murray TH. Guidelines for confidentiality in research on AIDS. *IRB: A Review on Human Subjects Research* 1984; 6(6): 1–7

Bove J. Transfusion-associated AIDS—A cause for concern. *N Engl J Med* 1984; 310(2): 115–116

Centers for Disease Control. An evaluation of the acquired immunodeficiency syndrome (AIDS) reported in health care personnel—United States. *Morb Mortal Wkly Rep* 1983; 32:358–360

Collins C, Sweeney T, Boring J et al. Undated

Curran J. AIDS—Two years later. *N Engl J Med* 1983; 309:610

Dubos R. *The Mirage of Health.* Harper and Row, New York, 1959

Golubjatnikov R, Pfister J, and Tillotson T. Homosexual promiscuity and the fear of AIDS. *Lancet.* 1983; 681

Judson F. Fear of AIDS and gonorrhea rates in homosexual men. *Lancet* Sept 17, 1983; 159–160

Krieger L. AIDS reporting code aims to protect privacy. *Am Med News* 1983; 26(37):20

Lieberson J. Anatomy of an epidemic. *New York Review of Books*, August 18, 1983, pp. 17–22

Marwick C. Confidentiality issues may cloud epidemiologic studies of AIDS. *J Am Med Assoc* 1983; 250(15): 1945

Odyssey of AIDS victim ends in death. *Am Med News* Nov 1983; p. 3

Rechy J. An exchange on AIDS. *New York Review of Books*, October 13, 1983, pp. 43–44

Weiss K. AIDS turmoil in the medical profession. *The New Physician* 1983; 32(6): 14, 16

### Chapter 12.  Immune System Modulation in AIDS Therapy

Ahuja K et al. Cimetidine as an immunomodulating agent in the AIDS syndrome. *J Allergy Clin Immunol* 1983; 71(1) Part 2:132

AIDS patients seeking alternative treatments. *Medical World News* Aug 22, 1983; pp. 8–9

Balfour HH et al. Acyclovir in immunocompromised patients with CMV disease: A controlled trial at one institution. Proceedings acyclovir symposium. *Am J Med* 1982; Vol. 73(1a) (Jul 20): 241–248

Bigar R et al. Thymosin alpha 1 levels and H/S ratio in homosexual men. *N Engl J Med* 1983; 309(1): 49

Bunby P. CMV vaccine work progressing. *J Am Med Assoc* 1983; 248(12)

Dardienne M and Safai B. Low serum thymic hormone levels in patients with AIDS. *N Engl J Med* 1983; 309(1): 48–49

Fryburg D, Rubinstein A, Reitura G, et al. Rationale for testing vitamin A as therapy for acquired immunodeficiency diseases. (Meeting abstract). *Fed Proc* 1984; 43(3): 606

Gelmann EP, Preble O, Steis R, et al. Treatment of Kaposi's sarcoma with alpha interferon. *Clin Res* 1984; 32(2): 415A

Gottlieb AA, Farmer JL, Hester RB, et al. Reconstitution of T-cell function in AIDS patients by use of leukocyte-derived endogenous immunomodulators. (Meeting abstract). *Clin Res* 1984; 32(2): 504A

Gottlieb MS, Hassner A, Fahey J, et al. Recombinant alpha-2 interferon therapy of acquired immunodeficiency syndrome in the absence of Kaposi's sarcoma. (Meeting abstract). *Clin Res* 1984; 32(2): 348A

Grieco MH, Reddy MM, Manvar D, et al. In-vivo immunomodulation by isoprinosine in patients with the acquired immunodeficiency syndrome and related complexes. *Ann Intern Med* 1984; 101(2): 206–207

Hersh EM, Reuben JM, Rios A, et al. Elevated serum thymosin alpha 1 levels associated with evidence of immune dysregulation in male homosexuals with a history of infectious disease of Kaposi's sarcoma. *N Engl J Med* 1983; 308(1)

Lane HC, Masur H, Long DL, et al. Immune reconstitution in the acquired immune deficiency syndrome. (Abstract) *Clin Res* 1983; 31:359

Lane HC, Masur H, Longo DL, et al. Partial immune reconstitution in a patient with the acquired immunodeficiency syndrome. *N Engl J Med* 1984; 311(17): 1099–1103

Lane HC, Masur H, Rook AH, et al. Treatment of patients with the acquired immunodeficiency syndrome with interleukin–2 or gamma interferon. (Meeting abstract). *Clin Res* 1984; 32(2): 351A

Linker C. Plasmapheresis in clinical medicine. *West J Med* 1983; 138(1): 60–69

Maheshwari RK, Sreevalsan T, Silverman RH, et al. Tunicamycin enhances the antiviral and anticellular activity of interferon. *Science* 1983; 219: 1339

Manvar D et al. Immunomodulation with isoprinosine in AIDS. *J Allergy Clin Immun* 1983; 71(1) pt. 2: 133

Marwick C. Interleukin II trial will try to spark flagging immunity of AIDS patients. *J Am Med Assoc* 1983; 250(9): 1125

Nishida J, Yoshikura H, Yoshida M, et al. Interferons inhibit fusion-forming ability of human T-cell leukemia virus. (Meeting abstract). *Clin Res* 1984; 32(2): 317A

Nose Y, Kambic HE, and Matsubura S. Introduction to therapeutic aphoresis. In *Plasmapheresis: Therapeutic Applications and New Techniques*, ed Nose Y, Malchesky LC, and Smith JW. Raven, New York, 1983

Osband ME, Cohen EB, Ho ZS, et al. Suppressin, a peptide that induces suppressor T cells: Identification, characterization and clinical results. (Meeting abstract). *Clin Res* 1984; 32(2): 355A

Oswald GA, Theodossi A, et al. Attempted immune stimulation in the "gay compromise syndrome." *Br Med J*. 1982; 285: 1082

Panem S. The emergent importance of lymphokines. *J Am Med Assoc* 1983; 249(2): 166–171

Pekarek RS et al. Abnormal cellular immune responses during acquired zinc deficiency. *Am J Clin Nutrition* 1979; 32: 1466

Plotkin SA et al. In vitro and in vivo responses of CMV to acyclovir. Proceedings acyclovir symposium. *Am J Med* 1982; Vol 73(1a) (Jul 20): 257–261

Preble O and Friedman RM. Interferon-induced alterations in cells: Relevance to viral and non-viral disease. *Lab Invest* 1983; 49(1): 4–18

Progress on AIDS slow as research and cases escalate. *Medical World News*, Nov 12, 1984, pp 30–32

Reddy MM et al. Indomethacin as an immunostimulant in AIDS. (Abstract). *Fed Proc* 1983; 42(4): 948

Rook AH, Masur H, Lane HC, et al. Interleukin II enhances the depressed natural killer and CMV specific activities of lymphocytes from patients with the AIDS. *J of Clin Invest* 1983; 72: 398–403

Serron B and Apesool D. Nutritional support and the immune system in cancer management. *Cancer Treatments Rep* 1981; 65 (Suppl 5): 115–120

Siegal BV and Morton JI. Vitamin C and the immune response. *Experentia* 1977; 33/315: 393

Siegel JN et al. T-cell suppression and contrasuppression induced by histamine H2 and H1 receptor agonists, respectively. *Proc Natl Acad Sci* (US) 1982; 79: 5052

Thomas ED. Bone marrow transplantation. *J Am Med Assoc* 1983; 249(18): 2528–2536

Tomar RH, Kloster BE, and Lamberson HV. Plasmapheresis increases $T_4$ lymphocytes in a patient with AIDS. *Am J Clin Patho* 1984; 81(4): 518–521

Tsang KY, Fudenberg HH, Koopman W, et al. Effect of isoprinosine on interleukin-2 (IL-2) production and TAC antigen bearing lymphocytes in vitro in patients with acquired immunodeficiency syndrome (AIDS). (Meeting abstract). *Clin Res* 1984; 32(2): 361A

## Chapter 14.  Preventing AIDS

Centers for Disease Control. Acquired immune deficiency syndrome (AIDS): Precautions for clinical and laboratory staffs. *Morb Mortal Wkly Rep* 1982; 31:577

————. Prevention of acquired immune deficiency syndrome (AIDS): Report of interagency recommendations. *Morb Mortal Wkly Rep* 1983; 32:101

## Chapter 15.  Psychological and Social Issues of AIDS and Strategies for Survival

Allison H, Gripton J, and Rodway M. Social work services as a component of palliative care with terminal cancer patients. In *Social Work in Health Care*. Haworth, New York, Summer 1983. 8(4): 30

Kastenbaum R. Death and development through the life span. In *New Meanings of Death*, ed. Feigel H. McGraw-Hill, New York, 1977, p 42

Kubler-Ross E. *On Death and Dying*. Macmillan, New York, 1969, p 5

# Index

and, 123–125; overview of,
122–123; patient dependency
and, 176–178; people with
AIDS and, 128–131; public
(government) money and, 131;
researchers and, 125–128; sexual activity and, 163; society and
resource allocation and, 131
Ethnic background, 17, 81; African
children with KS (Kaposi's sarcoma) and, 65, 71
Etoposide (VP-16), KS (Kaposi's
sarcoma) and, 68
Europe, 16
Excretions, caution and, 167, 168
Eyewear (protective), 198

Family: coping with AIDS and,
176–177, 189; fear of contagion
and, 172; home care and, 161–
164; lovers of gay patients as,
177–178, 183; support groups
and, 181–189
Fatigue, 37, 39
Fear: of contagion, 166, 175–176;
respiratory distress and, 154
Feces, 13
Fever, 36, 158, 192
Firemen, 171
First-aid personnel, 171
Food and Drug Administration, 19,
141
Food preparation, 162. *See also*
Nutrition
Friedland, Gerald, 13
Friedman, Alvin, 10
Funeral rites, 164; fear of con-
tagion and, 166. *See also* Death
Fungal infections, 62–63, 117

Gallo, Robert, 19, 72, 86

Gamma globulin, 103–104, 110
Garfield, Charles, 187
Gay bowel syndrome, 54. 78
Gay Men's Health Crisis (GMHC),
New York City, 184, 185–
186
Gay support groups, 184, 185–
189. *See also* Support
Gays. *See* Homosexuals (gays)
Genetic predisposition, 81, 83
Giardiasis, 55, 92
Gloves, wearing of, 173, 198
Goldstein, Dr., 140
Gonorrhea, 54, 94
Gordon, R. S., 114
Gottlieb, Michael, 10
Government: health insurance and,
182–183; resource allocation
and, 131; Social Security assis-
tance and, 181–182
Gowns, 198
Group therapy (AIDS Resource
Center), 187
Guilt, 178, 179

Haitians, 81; AIDS impact on,
97–98; case-control study and,
98–99; clinical manifestations
and, 91–93; epidemiology and,
90–91; etiology and, 93–94; as
high-risk group, 13–14, 113; immunology of AIDS and, 34; legal
risk factors and, 126; risk factor
among, 94–97; toxoplasmosis
and, 53
Hastings Center, 128
Haverkos, Harry, 13–14
Headaches, 39
Health care professionals, 165; CNS
(central nervous system) infections and, 156; conveying infec-

# Contributors

Victor Gong, MD. Editor. Clinical Instructor of Medicine, University of Medicine and Dentistry of New Jersey-Rutgers Medical School.

Leonard Calabrese, DO. Head, Section of Clinical Immunology, Department of Rheumatic and Immunologic Disease, Cleveland Clinic Foundation, Ohio. Clinical Consultant on The AIDS Task Force.

Keewhan Choi, PhD. Formerly Assistant Director, Division of Surveillance and Epidemiological Studies, Centers for Disease Control, Atlanta, Georgia.

Mary E. Cuff, RN, MA, CS. Clinical Instructor of Medicine, New York University Medical Center, New York.

Nirmal K. Fernando, MD. Assistant Professor of Infectious Disease, University of Medicine and Dentistry of New Jersey—Rutgers Medical School.

Benjamin Greer, MD. Department of Preventive Medicine, Stanford University, California.

Robert Hirsch, MD. Medical Director, Greater New York Blood Program, New York Blood Center, New York.

Peter Ho, MD. Until his untimely death from lymphoma, Dr. Peter Ho was with the Department of Infectious Disease, St. Michael's Medical Center, Newark, New Jersey.

Edward Johnson, MD. Assistant Director of Infectious Disease, Director of AIDS Clinic and AIDS hotline at St. Michael's Medical Center, New Jersey.

Virginia Lehman, MSW, ACSW. Department of Social Work, Bellevue Hospital Center, New York, affiliated with New York University School of Medicine.

Helen L. Lipscomb, PhD. Assistant Professor of Pathology and Laboratory Medicine, University of Nebraska Medical Center.

Michael Marsh, MD. Clinical Instructor of Medicine, University of Medicine and Dentistry of New Jersey-Rutgers Medical School.

Thomas H. Murray, PhD. Associate Professor, Ethics and Public Policy, Institute for the Medical Humanities, University of Texas Medical Branch, Galveston.

Michael Nissenblatt, MD. Assistant Clinical Professor of Oncology, University of Medicine and Dentistry of New Jersey-Rutgers Medical School.

Arye Rubinstein, MD. Professor of Pediatrics, Microbiology, and Immunology, Director of NIH AIDS Research Project, Albert Einstein College of Medicine, New York.

Noreen Russell, MSW, ACSW. Social Service Department, New York University School of Medicine, New York.

Leonard Scarpinato, DO. Department of Medicine, Cleveland Clinic Foundation, Ohio.

John W. Sensakovic, PhD., MD. Director of Nosocomial Disease Laboratory, Director Medical Education, St. Michael's Medical Center, Newark, New Jersey.

Daniel Shindler, MD. Assistant Professor of Medicine, University of Medicine and Dentistry of New Jersey-Rutgers Medical School.

Jeffrey Vieira, MD. Chief, Infectious Diseases Service, Brooklyn Hospital, New York.